Woman Who Glows in the Dark

Woman Who Glows in the Dark

A Curandera Reveals Traditional Aztec Secrets

of Physical and Spiritual Health

Elena Avila, R.N., M.S.N., *with Joy Parker*

Jeremy P. Tarcher/Putnam • a member of Penguin Putnam Inc. New York

Most Tarcher/Putnam books are available at special quantity discounts for bulk purchases for sales promotions, premiums, fund-raising, and educational needs. Special books or book excerpts also can be created to fit specific needs. For details, write Putnam Special Markets, 375 Hudson Street, New York, NY 10014.

Jeremy P. Tarcher/Putnam
a member of
Penguin Putnam Inc.
375 Hudson Street
New York, NY 10014
www.penguinputnam.com

Library of Congress Cataloging-in-Publication Data

Avila, Elena.
    Woman who glows in the dark: a curandera reveals
  traditional Aztec secrets of physical and spiritual health /
  Elena Avila with Joy Parker.
      p.   cm.
    ISBN 0-87477-958-8
    1. Magic.   2. Superstition.   I. Parker, Joy.
II. Title.
BF1615.A85   1999
615.8'52—dc21   98-36475 CIP

Printed in the United States of America
10   9   8   7   6   5   4   3   2   1

This book is printed on acid-free paper. ∞

Book design by Chris Welch

Acknowledgments

First, I would like to thank all of my teachers, past and present. A special thanks to my present teacher, Ehekateotl Kuauhtlinxan, for making me part of his family and for being a gentle teacher. To all the *comadritas* and *compadritos* from the Centro de Desarrollo Cultural Tetzkatlipoka Kallpulli, *gracias y Ometeotl*.

I wish to thank Rose Tarin, R.N., for telling me that I would make a good nurse. You opened the door to my destiny.

Words cannot express the gratitude I feel for all the clients who have had faith in me and my work. Your strong spirits and tenacity to heal continue to inspire me. You have been powerful teachers.

I eternally thank my students for their desire to accept curanderismo in their work. You are manifesting the elders' vision. My life has been enriched because I have been in circle with you. My life will circle yours always. I am not naming you individually, but you know who you are. *¡Que tengan una vida brillante!*

I wish to thank my family for encouraging me to write this book:

To my sister Rosario Martinez, who many years ago gave me a fancy pen for my book signings and has always been an *angelito* to me;

To my sister Irma Martinez, whose compassion and enthusiasm for all my new ventures gave me the courage to believe in myself;

To my sister Marta Gorges, for all of the adventures we had when we were kids;

To my brother Sergio Martinez, for your courage and strength. I cherish the dinner we shared in Lima, Peru;

To my brother-in-law Max Castillo, for being my *compadre* and for your silly jokes.

My appreciation to my beloved children is immense:

To Jamie Andres Avila, my firstborn, I thank you for accepting and loving me as I am. You are a good man and I honor your work in the movement against sexual assault and your acting. Like mother, like son;

To my only baby girl and fellow nurse, Sondra Susan Skory, I lovingly thank you for being a caring and fun daughter. I always look forward to our telephone chitchats. I honor your work as a pediatric intensive-care nurse and for being a great mom. I also thank you and my son-in-law John for my beloved grandchildren Samantha Nicole and Noah Christopher. I love it when they call me Mama Albuquerque;

I am forever grateful to Adrian Fernando Avila, my comedian son, who can always make me forget sadness by making me laugh. You have been one of my greatest teachers, *mijito;*

To my last-born, Abel Rene Avila, for your playfulness and strong spirit. I will never forget your wink when I spotted you among hundreds of your fellow Marines during your graduation. You make us proud. I thank you and Pam for giving me my beloved granddaughter Katherine Margaret Avila. Katie is my accomplice in play.

Thank you, *mijitos,* for choosing me to be your mom. I really love being your mom.

I am grateful to Kitty Farmer and her assistant Dana Roberts. Kitty is a caring agent, and because of her skill and love, my lecture tours are less stressful. If all else fails, I can always count on you and Dana;

To Clarissa Pinkola Estés, for being my friend and guardian angel. I feel that I am in the presence of someone very special when I see you or even talk to you on the phone. Your voice is soulful;

To Richard Prosapio, for reuniting me with nature;

To my friend Bernadette Vigil, for offering new dreams. Bernadette, you kept telling me, "Elena, write your book." I finally paid attention;

To Sabrina Garcia, for helping me through the dark times and for joining me in low-riding the feminist movement. We knew how to cruise;

To Jerry Mondragon, I love you for being my bro'. I thank you for being my writing partner for "Tu y Yo" and "Amantes Sin Casa." Some of my best times have been spent performing the plays and poetry I wrote with you. Thank you for all the times you stole me away from work and took me to the movies. Thank you for turning on my air conditioner and heater every year;

To Charlene Ortiz, *manita y comadre,* from the Center for Health Policy Development in San Antonio. You always believed in me. *Gracias;*

A special thanks to my *comadre* Malinalli, Ana Gutierrez Sisneros Mora. You taught me the true nature of humility. You have touched my heart;

Comadre Sandrea Gonzales, thank you for recommending me as Director of the Rape Crisis Center. I found a loyal friend when I met you;

To all my special friends in Taos. I love Taos and I love you.

Vicente Martinez, you are my special bro';

George and Beverly Chacon, your love for each other gives me hope;

Juanita Lavadie, thank you for the stories you shared about *luto;*

Linda Velarde, *gracias* for your unconditional love;

Flordemayo, what a treat to find another curandera in my neighborhood. You are a good friend. Thank you for the dreams you shared and the *pláticas* we got into;

To Andi Galicia, fellow nurse and my best friend from El Paso, I thank you for showing me so many healing paths all these years. Thank you for your grandmother's story on envy;

To Cris Phillips, I thank you for all the times you hugged me;

To my long-time friends Guillermo and Anneppe Ortiz and my beloved goddaughter Larena, who always provided a home for me in the Bay Area.

So many souls have helped shape my work and my life. I am eternally grateful. *Adelante mis valientes!*

My tender love to Jacinto-Temilotzin Sanchez. You pampered me
as I gave birth to the stories stored in my soul. When "Laughing
Flower" met "Warrior Poet," I found love. You are the one I finally
came home to.

Elena Avila

I would like to thank Joyce Fournier, Gene Stone, and all of my
friends at Morning Star Lodge who sat with me in ceremony and supported me with their prayers during the writing of this book.

My deepest gratitude goes to my dear friends:

Carol Basile and John Dickinson gave me valuable feedback on
this book and emotional support at every stage of the writing. You are
true friends of the soul.

Leslie Baer was a constant source of inspiration, confidence, and
strength. Through the many years of work you have done with your
humanitarian organization Xela-Aid in Quetzaltenango and outlying
Mayan villages, you have been able to give me much valuable advice
about keeping safe in Guatemala. I also thank you for setting up a
meeting between me and Amalia Vasquez, master weaver, midwife,
and head woman of the village San Martín Chiquito, a friendship that
has lasted to this day.

I wish to honor all those who have taken me by the hand in the last
ten years and taught me about indigenous cultures, their history, and
their healing arts. Your help and friendship prepared me for the writing of this book in ways that no amount of "research" ever could have
done.

Heartfelt thanks to David Friedel and the late, great Linda Schele,
who brought me into the world of the Mayans as we wrote two books
together.

Much gratitude to my friends Malidoma and Sobonfu Somé, who
gave me so many gifts from the culture of the Dagara in Africa.

And thirteen thank-yous to Tzutujil Mayan shaman Martín Prechtel, for sharing so much with me about the nature of healing and being
called to walk the healing path.

Many thanks to the apprentice curanderas for the stories they so
willingly shared with me in the preparation of chapters 6 and 7. While
space did not allow us to use all of your beautiful and profound experiences, your generous help served only to deepen my understanding

of curanderismo. I am also grateful for your companionship on our trip to Guatemala.

Special thanks go to Valerie Berg, who booked transportation and accommodations for us in Guatemala, allowed us to stay in her home our first night, and served us a heavenly meal.

I also wish to acknowledge the deep wisdom of my mother, Helen Parker, who was always willing to listen and comfort me when I felt tired or discouraged.

Last, this book could not have been written without the steadfast love of my sister, Debra Jurich, who always gave me her ear and her sound counsel.

Joy Parker

We both would like to express our heartfelt thanks to Jeremy P. Tarcher, who had the vision to see the value of a book on curanderismo and brought the two of us together to write it. Without your help, this wonderful adventure that we have shared would not have been possible.

We also would like to thank literary agent Elaine Markson, who not only negotiated a wonderful contract but helped us all along the rocky road from idea to finished product. We are grateful for your sensitivity, tact, creative spirit, and heartfelt support. You are a great and dear lady.

Thanks to publisher Joel Fotinos, who made it possible for us to travel throughout Guatemala and Mexico doing important research for this book.

Much gratitude to our editor, Wendy Hubbert, who helped to shape our vision and constantly challenged us to be our best. We owe you deep thanks for your belief in this book and your continued work to give it a home in the world.

We also wish to thank editorial assistant Jocelyn Wright, for shepherding this book through its many stages, and always being available to answer our questions.

Gratitude to our copy editor, Deborah Miller, who was unfailing in her diligence, checking all of the difficult spellings of the Nahuatl language, and helping us to clarify our prose.

Joy Parker and Elena Avila

This book is dedicated to Coyolxauhqui,
Mother Who Glows in the Dark,
and in loving memory of my parents,
Matias G. Martinez and Ada Brito Martinez,
and to my sisters Laura and Sonia.
— ELENA AVILA

To Frank Parker, loving father
— JOY PARKER

Woman Who Glows in the Dark

I woke up to my illusions,
And now I can't sleep.

I have no desires,
and now I can't eat . . .
what you dish out to me.

I'll stay awake forever if
    I have to.

I live in the crack of an egg —
in the space between galaxies
and earth mud.
Along the thin borders
of enlightenment and
darkness.

I saw through the smoky mirror,
and my third eye winked at me!

Time is an illusion,
and eternity lives
in the cracks of everything
that is dualized.

I like living
in the middle of
either/or,
and gray is my color
in black/white.
I'm cozy in the nucleus
of past/future and . . .

I am the ember seed in
light/dark.
I am
Woman who glows in the dark.

I'll stay awake forever
       if I have to.

—Elena Avila

Contents

Introduction

Beginning in childhood, many are urged and taught by their cultures to not see too much. One should certainly not dare to call oneself artist or poet. One must agree to agree, even though strongly sensing otherwise, that only things which have their atoms packed together so tightly that they are able to be seen by the egos of all—that these are the only things that ought to matter in life.

But in curanderismo, it is just the opposite. The mother tongue is poetics. The healer is an artist. The invisible worlds are palpably felt and acknowledged directly along with the consensual reality.

Too much time spent in an injection-molded plasticizing culture means that one must swerve every day, and hard, against being absorbed by a learned blindness to the interior life. But for many, a weakening of sight, a dropping of the hands, a kind of nonrighteous surrender insinuates itself anyway.

Pressure to conform for scant reward, and/or threats of marginalization because of one's beliefs, may force an individual to attempt to assimilate into this least layer of culture, thereby causing one's relationship to all things to slowly become defective. There, one becomes disconnected from the observable essence, from the affecting vitality of all things. It is not supposed to be this way for humans. Relationship to all matters and aspects of the world is meant to be complementary, wherein one is able to feel the electricity, and the condition of that electricity, inside of all things.

Much of our literature regarding various phenomena of spirit, mind, body, rite and ritual of all sorts, whether in art, sociology, anthropology, culture, or science, is too often laid down with either a stupefying giddiness accompanied by claims that cannot be justified, or else validly described, but devoid of a true élan vital. These cause detached—as in detached retina—observations, instead of clear and useful observations.

For instance, an observer, surely good-hearted but also without in-depth comprehension, might say that "at the center of curanderismo is la curandera; the healer who intervenes, the one who asks for intercession, who praises and reweaves the unraveled worlds of mind, body, and spirit in order to improve the mundane and spiritual health of the patient." Such an observation, however, would be in grave error.

Truly at the center, firstly and lastly, is the flower-bedecked God, called and accompanied by the drum, or by the embers of copal incense burning with piercing fragrance, and/or by the white smoke twirling upward from hundreds of sweet-smelling wax candles all ablaze. The phrase "New Age" has never been and will never be a part of curanderismo. God is the exact center, the precise mother drum of the entire relationship we call curanderismo. That this is so can only be realized by observation through eyes that are clear, not hooded, those that are filled with the kind of un-knowing that desires nevertheless, to learn, rather than from an unknowing that cares little for the inextinguishable heart of a thing.

Down through the centuries, there have been myriad efforts to describe what I would call *el aliento profundemente*, the great breath to be found in the art of the healer. In a proper world, description itself is a phenomenon which carries a high degree of numinousness in the right hands. Though some few portraits of certain aspects of curanderismo, such as those beautifully detailed and translated in the Popul Vuh, the great Mayan holy book, have been painterly and shapely, others have used flat, muddied pigments that caused the vis-age of the whole to be destroyed rather than to be described in all its nuances and splendor.

The following are examples of further distortions of curan-derismo. I do not cite them as condemnations, but only as examples of a typical kind of overpainting that has occurred for eons and which now must be carefully removed in order for the true face of curanderismo underneath to be revealed accurately and beautifully.

According to what once was considered a stylish second- and third-order analysis, that is, an attempted ratiocination of the phenomenon from the outside rather than from the inside, curanderismo might be described as: "A folkway associated with a certain ethnic group, particularly those from the lower classes in various of the lands now called Old Mexico."

It might be said further that "such people believe that God is delivered into the healer, so that individuals so designated may then perform an eccentric set of rites while pronouncing certain proscribed words. Various artifacts are burned and/or fanned in various ways, after which the patient is declared 'cured.' The patient pays the curandera with a previously agreed upon currency, and after that, all life returns to normal."

¡Ay! No. In such a portrayal, the crucial insights into the mysteries of healing are missing completely. Surely a massacre of all the poets in the world would have had to take place for God to agree to be pleased with such a "heart-nailed-shut" story. When describing artfulness, resorting to reductionistic narratives is rather like describing a tiger leaping with all its claws spread and glinting as simply "a striped hide flung into the air, the mass of which appears to be larger at one end than at the other." This kind of description is not any kind of living *ology,* study of, or knowing. Flat writing is taxidermy.

Consider for a moment an alternative notion like the next, similarly used to describe the religious rites of Haitians,

Santo Domingians, Hawaiians, American Indians, Aztecas, and others struck down and colonized. "Curanderismo is the devil's work. It is carried out by the demon-possessed, who are really, in effect, complete quacks. Their prayers, exhortations, dancings are of a nature that is ungodly. They are heathens; they are shams."

¡Double and triple ay! More than a thousand times, no! *Dio mio, mio Dio,* where in such a report is the One who is central to many faiths; in much curanderismo, also called *El Cristo,* the Lord of Love? The writer, like a madman haircutter, has also sheared away all presence of His mother, Our Beautiful Lady, *la nuestra señora,* Guadalupe.

Other erroneous or flattened-out descriptions similar to all the above can be found many times over in diaries as ancient as those of the sixteenth-century Spanish conquistador Bernal Diaz, and as recently as this year's journal articles written by any J. Doe who claims that anything outside his or her own purview ought be considered alarmingly senseless and outré. To my mind, no one can write vividly or validly about the interior life of the spirit unless they *live* there —live there truly, not as tourists, not as visitors, not as developers, but as authentic citizens.

It is a good thing then, that despite detractors, haters, and marauders, nothing can be lost forever that has been loved forever. Throughout the world there continue to live numerous souls who still are attached to the ancestral roots they derive from. They continue to blast away centuries of scorn, predation, and manifest-destiny projections onto their deep and godly understandings and rituals. The Latinos of the world continue, over the centuries, to meld their religious rites that are, in part, Old World, and in part, New World

Católico. Curanderismo is a part of the great colorful weaving that results.

I have, in my older years now, come to chuckle at many things I once used to only ponder darkly, or else in some bewilderment. One of the popular cultural tenets I find mirth in now is the popular idea that psychology began with Freud one hundred years ago. It is true that Freud was in many ways a sensitive observer, and Jung also, but think on this: The word *psychology* means, literally, the study of the life of the soul. The word *psyche* is derived from the ancient word *prushke,* which is related to both the image of *la mariposa,* the butterfly, and *la alma,* the soul. The word is also related to the essence of the breath; in other words, to the animating force without which all of us would lie dead upon the ground. *Psychology* in its truest sense is not the study of behavior per se, but the study of the animating force. The same is so in curanderismo.

In this manner, psychology began unfolding millions of years ago. It is ancient. It first rose not from the elegant thinking of the bow-tie and cravat tribes, but from under the wild locks of those who thought they could enter the mind of an eagle, those who affably hailed the bruins they met upon the path, those who dressed like a scatter of crows, those who could replicate exactly the howl of the now extinct dire wolf.

To the strictly Western mind, this sounds somewhat eerie, I know. But it is not odd if one has the talent for it. Think of how we marvel over those whose talents are to be found in painting and sculpture, or in engineering and physics. *That* is the same kind of respect the elders of the Mexicano families teach to their children with regard to those who possess the gifts of entering, healing, and translating spirit-to-spirit, soul-to-soul.

Curanderismo deals, as do certain psychoanalytic theories, with the negative and positive principles of the psyche. Curanderismo goes much further, however. One takes into account not only the stories of a person's life, the psyche's dreams, the mundane situation, but also, in investigating the life of the soul in depth, one prays over the person. The prayers are for vision, for strength and for wholeness, meaning a kind of rememberedness. In curanderismo, dreams *do* offer assistance and direction. At depth, in the psyche, one experiences that the inner and outer worlds *do* leak into one another.

In psychoanalysis, we say that mastery of the interior world and the exterior world is dependent on not growing one-sided. For, if one does, the roots of the person, by virtue of the weight of their one-sidedness, will pull loose from the ground that holds the very things we desire most in life; intelligent meaning, unfolding talents, practice of compassion and love, the animating spirit.

The relationship between curandera and *alma*, patient, does not end when the rite/analysis is over, or when *la quenta*, the bill, has been paid. The greatest curanderas and curanderos keep the *velas* burning for each soul's health for months, years, often forever.

Curanderismo, like classical Jungian psychoanalysis, takes into account that a modern person is often well and properly socialized in early life, but also in some ways deeply misled; that the person is often wrongly encouraged, rewarded and even threatened into living a life that excludes an entire continent of knowledge—the life of the soul.

Like psychoanalysis, curanderismo has an interplay with the processes of the collective unconscious. Notice I said *processes*. One of the errors a neophyte might make is to think that it is the collective unconscious itself that is so interesting. No, looking into the collective unconscious by intellect alone, and even with much affection, is still like looking at fascinating relics in a glass case in a museum. Rather, it is *the processes, not the representations,* of the collective unconscious that affect us, that cause one's *vida imprescindible,* vitality of life, to remain truly alive, properly capable of offering both meaning and direction.

This is not to say that psychoanalysis is curanderismo, or that curanderismo is psychoanalysis, for neither is the other, and each has very different healing pathways and trainings. The training to be a psychoanalyst is far shorter than the training for being a curandera—about eight years in a program certified by the father-house in Zurich, as compared to about fifty years, or more, of practice in curanderismo.

Though both have distinguished boundaries, most of their methods and their ideations are not shared in common. But what is similar is that both rely on encouraging the movement of the psyche toward a more integral viewpoint, one that provides additional and symbolic information and formations, ones that assist not a life spent on the sleeping couch or in front of the TV, but a life of strength, a life of creation, a life striving toward *las beatitudes,* the septet of beautiful blessednesses.

So, shall we assign blame for muffling the signals from the interior world to the cruel and creepy hands of a misguided culture, or to observers' flattened-out reports that seem to encourage a portion of the great collective to continue its

contempt for the interior and sacred life? Is it not the fault of
the tremendously degraded burlesque that has come to dom-
inate the rank and suppurating barrens of too much of the Internet, television media, film carcasses, and *los políticos
solomente,* "politicians' voices only," airwaves?

No, in the end, it is none of these, *in essence.* They are mere
contributors to the offal piles of the centuries. What? What
are you saying? Surely these are at the bottom of it? No.
There are others who are far more responsible. The reasons
that the soul is so often treated poorly in the larger culture,
the reason that it is so often dishonored and pointed to as a
pathetic, poor, strangled thing is because so many individuals
do not say aloud, and do not live out loud, their absolutely
certain knowledge of the soul.

They try, instead, to keep the interior life "a private affair,"
tying themselves into knots in order to try to live an outer life
as though the world of angels and messengers, random evil
and redeeming love, helpers and inspiratrices did not exist.

This is what causes the state of soul to be degraded in culture. Though it can be understood that no person has a particularly deep desire to be tormented, misunderstood, or
ridiculed for his or her interior knowledge, when we do fear
so much that we turn into know-nothing cardboard cut-outs,
then a terrible peril is engendered: The life of the soul writ
large as it ought to be in culture withers away instead.

If there is one thing that the faithful people of all deep and
ancient creeds believe—this being also definitely so amongst
we who are *Católicas y Mexican-Americans*—it is that faith has
no timbre and no strength unless . . . that it is no faith at all,
unless one lives it out publicly.

This does not mean jabbering about it incessantly, but

neither does it mean denying that one follows a wild and precious soul life—one that helps to keep the lanterns lit high enough to see by, during dark times in one's own life and in the lives of others.

Without the daily interaction with interior and exterior worlds, though one may feel made safe from being shaken about by others, in interacting with only the outer world with no support from the inner, one falls into a shaking sickness anyway. Sick from lack of passion, and shaking from lack of meaningful animation. One's soul becomes afflicted by being mistreated so. One day, it may just simply walk away from its person.

Then, the poor person left behind feels deadened, feels ennui, frustration, feels agitated, but cannot realize the source. But the curanderas know why. It is an issue of the person's ignorance about what constitutes *la vida verdad*, true life. What is said to be missing is the reality of the world of spirit and that body of wisdom about godliness that directly touches, leads, prods, and saves a human being from a false selfhood, from a life of deadening choices. This is what curanderismo is so much concerned with: assisting the One, who, when spotting the child soul stranded and frightened at the edges of raging waters, lifts her across with holy and invisible hands. That One. It is that One of whom we speak.

There are essentially two aspects to the disturbance of one-sidedness: undervaluation and overvaluation. The latter attitude is as destructive as the former. Overvaluation occurs when the psyche of an individual, often starved of spirit and meaning, launches into a headfirst and reckless leap into thinking that curanderismo and/or the life of the interior is the be-all and end-all. Having lost touch with earth, their shoes now dangling out of the clouds, they are no longer good for anything.

Curanderismo is *practical and of spirit both*. It is meant to be, and must be this way. What is godly is understood and enjoyed in a dancing way whenever possible, but also, such must be carried out into the world and applied pragmatically to every aspect of life.

The error of jumping into the divine without sounding or concern is somewhat like a goat with an aimless wanderlust who has just discovered a blackberry bush (but forgotten the bush has thorns). This has never been effective for long. Why? Because the essence of the divine is realized by longing, and cannot be learnt in the midst of greedy enthusiasm. That kind of hubris in one who is too ready, willing, and able to say that this one way, this one path is everything, that there is no other, and that the acolyte is pre-ordained to just know that it is so for them—is not the way. Again, no. This one does not know anything. And that is what is dangerous. Not knowing the limits. One is not supposed to gobble up curanderismo, but to find nourishment in being *of* its essence: God.

Something must be said here too, for the sake of cautioning the naive to avoid those who are sometimes called *los estomagos vacios*, the empty ones, those who take on the stripe and rattle of the holy inauthentically, without doing the very hard and very long work required, and who often, unfortunately, make claims to power they do not truly possess. Whether *curandera, cantadora, partera*, midwife, *sobadora*, masseuse, or any of the other categories of kinds of curanderas—the healer is forever in direct training, is never "graduated or matriculated." The helpful arts of curanderismo are not something one can purposely set out to master, the way one goes to school. It cannot be learned without a complete and spoken agreement between the living soul of *la maestra o el maestro* and the living soul of the other. The exchange, and it *is* a true exchange between both, is often made in the kitchen or in the side dirt yard, or in a tiny room, or under an enormous sky. It cannot be learned by traveling to far places for a while, nor by hanging out with, nor by simply learning the language of, nor by collecting experiences of ritual as souvenir. This is why there is no terminal degree granted in curanderismo. Quite the contrary. Every curandera, *partera, sobadora,* remains forever an apprentice, that is, a servant for, and to, all blessed life.

In curanderismo, it is taught that insight is strengthened by climbing the mountain of one's own humility. The curandera strives toward this constantly. Falling down, getting back up. Falling down again, running to catch up and hold on again. It is not easy. And what is humility? In curanderismo, it is allowing not oneself but God to take the center place.

In part because la curandera is not a vehement seeker of limelight, and does not normally perform demonstrations at Madison Square Garden, but rather in solitude, in his or her own community bounded by the heart, there are not thousands of treatises on curanderismo. I hope there will never be, for though curanderismo is a common enactment, it is as yet a rare thing to behold—like glimpsing a ruby-throated hummingbird—one of the *autografías* of *Tonanzin*—or stumbling across the rare blue columbines high up at misty timberline in the Rockies.

But, too, truth be known, many of us have spoken amongst ourselves for decades now about the necessity of bringing out more of our work to the larger culture, facing squarely the ramifications of doing so—so that *our* culture can be known as it truly is, and *in our own voices,* but equally so, in service of compassion for the sake of a poor world that we assess could perhaps mindlessly, accidentally, and irrevocably catapult itself into its endtimes. So much of the world and many of its people seem to be suffering faster, harder, far more mightily than ever before. We hear. We want to respond.

This book, *Woman Who Glows in the Dark,* is in the vanguard of just such a compassionate action toward the world. Because we have very few detailed texts from true curanderas, most of whom until very recently, but also continuing, were, and are, non-literate, it is an excellent thing that Elena Avila has agreed to tell the story of her unique ways, her interesting life, her eye-witness practice as la curandera.

In her book is the beginning of a history of curanderismo. The content, because it has most often been hidden from the view of most, may seem, at first, somewhat unfamiliar. This is good, for it means that to this point, curanderismo has remained well protected, and also hidden away for the most part, from glittering eyes, trivializations and corruptions. It is my hope and prayer that it will remain so sheltered by all who learn of it.

It is on a horizon line of rare sightings that Elena Avila's book stands. Her work and life form a prototype. Hers is a heretofore hidden treasure that she is capable of relating to us in both academic voice and in the voice of poet. Here, she demonstrates her tremendously generous nature, her patience and willingness to tell the whole story. Her deep and many years' long commitment to this practice has earned her many honors, as is right and proper. But more so, being a curandera is a solitary, wise, wounding, returning-from-the-dead kind of life and cycle—one that she has agreed to, and has engaged in, not for just one year, or from time to time, not for just two years out of ten years, but for decades. You will see as you read that it is through her true sorrows and her true times—as my grandmother used to sing, *lo lo contento,* of contentment and tranquility—of verily *being,* that she has grown into a fierce lover to, and defender of, the soul.

Elena Avila, like those I have loved most, is at the same time deeply Old World and also gaily New World. I first met her in the desert under a very low, glowering sunset. Her little house in northern New Mexico was just a few miles down the rutted road from a *rez* casino sign that was in overkill with its thousands of lightbulbs stuttering. At Elena's invitation, I parked my old, low-slung black car on her front lawn just "like any decent Chicana." I knew from this alone that we would become fast friends.

In our time, we have heard much from the Eastern wisdom tradition, and much, much from Western wisdom tradition, and also from the Northern wisdom traditions of the Indians. Now, I invite you to read also about a pure and authentic Southern wisdom tradition, curanderismo, well described by La Elena, a curandera *superfina,* one who lives on the *inside* of the phenomenon, one whose roots are in the rich, dark soil of the true work, one who knows the fragrant Center utterly.

You are in good hands.

Clarissa Pinkola Estés, Ph.D.
poet, psychoanalyst, *cantadora*
Cheyenne, Wyoming
October 1998

In the Beginning

Five hundred years ago a new medicine began to evolve on this continent, what I call the medicine of the "three-headed serpent," the blending together of the people, medicine, and hearts of three cultures. It began when the Spaniards arrived in the New World and met up with the spiritual, earth-oriented medical practices of the indigenous people of Mexico and what is now the southwestern United States. At the time, the Spaniards had an advanced system of healing that incorporated herbology as well as the concept that the body has four "humors," blood, phlegm, yellow bile, and black bile. These humors were further subdivided into the dualities of "wet and dry" and "hot and cold," a system of classifying illness and wellness.

Spanish medicine met up with systems such as the Aztec *Wewepahtli* (Greatest Medicine), which had a profound and complex understanding of the healing and maintenance of the body, soul, spirit, and emotions. This medicine, called *curanderismo*, continued to evolve after the Spaniards imported African slaves who practiced their own complex, ancient, sophisticated spirituality and healing modalities. As the three cultures intermixed and a new blend of people, the mestizos, was born, a new "medicine of the people" began to evolve, a system that was deeply rooted in practical observation, in the thousand-year-old traditions of three continents, and in the personal style, creativity, intuition, and spiritual strength of the healer.

Curanderismo comes from the Spanish word *cura*, which means "to heal" or "to be a priest." In the lectures and workshops that I give across the country, I stress that one of the most important aspects of curanderismo is that it does not separate the soul and spirit from the body. It is medicine and spirituality practiced simultaneously. Only recently has traditional Western medicine come to understand the importance of this concept. In 1994, only three out of 120 medical schools in the U.S. offered courses devoted to exploring the role of spiritual belief and prayer in healing. By 1998, approximately forty medical schools began to develop courses in this area. In curanderismo, there has never been a severing between the emotional, physical, mental, and spiritual totality that

makes up a person. There is no separation between the nature of humans and their environment. The folk healer does
not withhold her own religious and spiritual beliefs apart
from her treatments. In curanderismo, the healing takes place
under one roof, with earth as the foundation and God as the
source.

Curanderismo's strength comes from its practice of always
incorporating whatever is useful and available into its treatments, in an intuitive and creative way. A modern medical
doctor must go through a procedural manual, but curanderismo uses whatever works: herbs, counseling, soul retrieval, psychodrama, rituals, spiritual cleansings—and, yes,
referrals to medical doctors. As a curandera and a trained
psychiatric nurse, I find that I heal most effectively when I
combine my medical knowledge with my instincts and divine
guidance. I have dressed women in men's clothing to help
them to get in touch with the masculine side of their nature. I
have taken my patients for long walks in the desert to prepare
them for *limpias* (spiritual cleansings). If a massage is needed
to help a client unburden himself of his troubles, I have him
lie down on my massage table, and I work with him until his
heart opens up and the words come out. I take patients on
trance journeys, accompanied by drumming, to find lost parts
of their soul. I give my clients homework, asking them to
keep a journal, to bring in pictures of their family or partners
to help in healing from a relationship that has ended or is in
serious trouble. I have taken people to graveyards to mourn
their dead and recover their grieving souls. I have blessed
marriages, and I have also helped people to let go of relationships with love and forgiveness when divorce is inevitable.

People from every walk of life have come through the door

of my treatment room: doctors, Navajo grandmothers, lawyers, social workers, blue-collar workers, Catholics, Africans, housewives, psychologists, Chicanos, Anglos, and people of Asian and African descent. Over the last twenty-three years, I have seen almost every kind of physical, spiritual, and emotional illness imaginable. The altar in my treatment room holds symbols of many different spiritual belief systems: Catholic, Aztec, Mayan, North Native American.

When I talk to people about curanderismo, I often compare it to a traditional Mexican dessert known as *capirotada*, a wonderful bread pudding made during Lent. Like curanderismo, this pudding uses everything in its making. My mother made a delicious *capirotada* using a recipe that was passed down from her mother. You use bread (or flour tortillas if you don't have bread), cheddar cheese (but longhorn cheese will do), *piloncillo* (if you cannot get *piloncillo*, use brown sugar). If you are out of brown sugar, use white sugar. You also use raisins, tiny sprinkles of different colored candies, and piñon nuts (if you are from New Mexico). You can add chopped pecans if you are from Texas, California, or Mexico, plus cinnamon, butter, cream, or whatever else your mother taught you to add to the *capirotada*.

As a curandera, I not only use whatever is available, practical, and creative in my practice, but I also individualize my treatments. This is because I know that the same disease found in two different people may need to be treated in two different ways because the individuals are different. Their energy bodies, past and present experiences, temperaments, and souls are different. The expert on any condition is always the person living with that condition. Labeling or getting too attached to a diagnosis made by a medical practitioner or a curandera will close the person's creative forces of healing. Every illness has its story, and the job of the healer is to uncover that story.

A Curandera's Concept of Medicine and Wellness

Curanderismo is an earthy, natural, grounded health-care system that seeks to keep all of the elements of our being in balance. Curanderos believe that human beings—along with animals, plants, minerals, water, earth, air, and fire—are a part of the living earth system. Illness occurs when one does not live in harmony with all aspects of self and nature.

Curanderos believe that it is not enough to heal the body. One must heal the wounded soul as well. When a person is raped, or injured in an automobile accident, or a woman has an abortion, the physical scars might go away, but the scars on the soul do not. Trauma causes a part of the soul to get frightened and run away into hiding. When this happens, a part of our energy is no longer accessible to us. We need 100 percent of our soul's energy to be in good physical, mental, and spiritual health.

A soul that is off balance is said to be suffering from *susto,* and the treatment involves a "soul retrieval." If one's spirit has lost faith in God or the divine, one suffers an illness as real as a physical or mental illness. All aspects of the self suffer, and one will experience diseases that affect one's body, mind, emotions, spirits, soul, family, community, and nature. The curandera understands this concept of illness and has a knowledge of how to guide the patient back to balance.

Since many of my clients are women, I have also developed special insights into women's health care in my practice. Curanderismo lends itself effectively to dealing with women's health issues, both physical and emotional. I have helped women to heal from the emotional scars of abortion, the physical and emotional challenges of menopause, eating disorders, the trauma of rape, and the psychological scars of childhood and spousal abuse. Since women tend to see the world more in terms of relationships than do men, many of their physical maladies have a basis in the stress they feel when a relationship with a spouse, partner, child, friend, or coworker becomes unbalanced or toxic. Curanderismo provides many tools for healing or giving closure to relationships: *limpias*, *pláticas*, and ceremonies for soul retrieval and the healing of the heart.

Curanderas have insights into the way a patient perceives her own illness within the context of her personal values, family, and culture. No treatment goal can be envisioned that does not take these beliefs into consideration. No matter who we are, we all retain cultural values, at times without realizing it. For example, one of the first questions I ask a new client is what kind of spiritual belief system she follows. If my patient is a seventy-year-old Catholic grandmother, I draw her attention to the images of Jesus and the Virgin Mary on my altar. I don't intimidate her by lecturing to her about Aztec philosophies of spirit and soul. If my client is an Anglo lawyer who does not feel comfortable about personifying God, I talk about divine or universal energy. If the patient is a woman who is uncomfortable with masculine concepts of divinity, we might talk about the three images that are painted on the screen behind my altar, the Virgin of

Guadalupe, the Moon, and Coyolxauhqui, the Aztec Cosmic
Mother.

Many times I have had Chicano families come to me complaining of a curse that was laid on a son, daughter, mother,
or father. Although I do not believe in curses, I respect the
cultural perspective of those who do, and I listen to them
with respect. Part of a cure, however, involves accurately
identifying the cause of the physical or emotional illness in
language that makes sense to the patient. Sometimes the
"cursed" individual is suffering from some kind of chemical
imbalance, such as schizophrenia, and needs medication and
psychiatric help. Sometimes a soul retrieval is the best treatment. Sometimes there is a physical problem that can be
cleared up by a medical doctor. Curanderas help to build up
a person's energy system and self-esteem, and teach him or
her how to break the vicious cycle of depression and hopelessness.

Many people who come to me fear that God is punishing
them with illness or bad luck because they have done something wrong. I tell them that God does not make us sick, we get
sick because we do not take care of ourselves, or because we
inherit an illness, or because of aging, or because the atmosphere is carrying an energy our body cannot resist (viruses,
bacteria). Our bodies can only take us so far.

In the West, especially since the development of wonder
drugs such as penicillin and advanced medical technologies
such as organ transplants and MRIs, we have spent the past
several decades believing that science can heal us. Finally we
have come full circle and begun to look back toward our past
and toward those cultures that have preserved their holistic,
nature-based healing traditions. People are beginning to real-

ize that science and technology cannot provide all the answers in the healing profession.

The Roots of Curanderismo

African Medicine

Millions of African slaves came to America and Mexico between 1500 and 1870, bringing spiritual beliefs and medical
practices that were incorporated into curanderismo. This is
not surprising, because these Africans had many things in
common with the Native Americans of the New World. Both
practiced an earth-oriented spirituality that saw the world as
alive and inhabited by spiritual energies with which they
could interact through ceremony, offerings, and prayer. Both
saw soul and spirit not as something holy and disconnected
from the body, as the Spaniards did, but as inside of us,
grounded in our physical body, emotions, and mind.

In his book *Of Water and the Spirit,* West African medicine
man Malidoma Somé writes about the healing traditions and
belief systems that his people have practiced for thousands of
years. When I read this book, I found many things that reminded me of the beliefs that underlie curanderismo, beliefs
that, no doubt, were brought to America and Mexico by the
slaves who came from West Africa. One of the most important concepts that our two traditions share is that of community. For both traditions, health is connected to community
because community serves as a link to an individual's sense of
identity, meaning, and purpose. Both cultures also believe
that emotional, physical, and spiritual health depend on a
healthy relationship with the ancestors. Somé's tribe, the Da-

gara, have many ceremonies and rituals in which the ancestors are honored and petitioned. In my healing practices, I always do the same. In fact, one of Mexico's most important
holidays is the Day of the Dead, in which graves are dressed
with flowers and food offerings, and the dead are honored
with altars in the home.

There are many other similarities between my culture and
Somé's. Both possess a rich storytelling tradition that helps in
healing. Both believe in the connection between thought and
reality, between healing and nature, and both have a concept
of the spirit as that part of us that protects the soul. Both see
animals, plants, and all living things as our brothers and sisters. As a curandera, I use ritual, ceremonies, dances, drums,
rattles, divinations, painting of the face and body during ceremony, and fasting as tools for healing. So does Somé's tribe.
Both cultures see the soul as something that can be lost, and
the health of the soul as a crucial factor in the health of the
person.

Most traditional African homes have an altar, and curanderos likewise use altars as an important part of their work.
Both traditions honor the elders, and maintain a tradition of
passing on the medicine to a chosen apprentice when the time
is right.

Both Dagara medicine and curanderismo see the earth as a
place of healing and transformation. During initiation, the elders of Malidoma's tribe ask young boys to bury one another
in the earth to help them in their initiatory transformations.
One of my Aztec teachers, Andres Segura, taught me to do
the same thing for women who had been raped and needed to
be healed and grounded.

When I do a healing for someone from Africa, it is not surprising that he or she feels comfortable with my tools and methods. Several years ago, an African man who was living in America called me up and asked for a healing. He was going through many difficulties adjusting to life in this country, and a friend suggested that he get a *limpia* from me. When we met, the African man was honest and told me that he was not familiar with curanderismo, but that he was desperate and needed to feel his spirit again. He had heard good things about me and was willing to give my methods a try. I gave him a spiritual cleansing, which included a ritual to the five directions, and when we finished his face was glowing. He thanked me profusely and he told me, "Your *limpia* is so similar to our curing of the spirit. I have finally found something that makes me feel at home."

When I remember his words, I think we are very fortunate that African medicine was one of the ingredients that went into the wonderful *capirotada* pudding of curanderismo. Its gifts came to us, born out of the will and strength of the African soul and spirit to survive in the New World. A strong spirit is very difficult to kill, and I thank my African brothers and sisters for their contribution to curanderismo. My ancestors and the ancestors of my African brothers and sisters are very pleased.

Spanish Medicine

When the Spanish came to the new world in the fifteenth century, they had one of the most highly regarded medical systems available in the Western world. Their medicine was an eclectic combination of the Greek and Roman practices of Hippocrates and of the Arabic medicine and health practices handed down by the Moors. This system was complemented by Judeo-Christian religious symbols and rituals, and medieval European witchcraft. Spanish medical knowledge was organized into two very well defined theories: the rational and the spiritual.

The Rational Theory. The rational approach was introduced into Spain by the Moors and had its roots in the medical theories of the ancient Greek physicians Galen and Hippocrates, and of the Chinese physician Ho. This medical approach was based upon a system of "humors." Within the Greek theory of humors, the human body is composed of four elements— black bile, yellow bile, blood, and phlegm—and each humor was believed to have its own "complexion." Black bile caused melancholy, and its characteristics were cold and dry. Yellow bile caused bad temper, and its characteristics were hot and dry. The humor known as blood was hot and wet, and phlegm was cold and wet. Mental or physical sickness developed when one of these humors was not in perfect equilibrium with all the others, and it was the healer's job to ascertain the imbalance of humors and correct it. A good example in curanderismo is *bilis* (rage), a hot and dry condition caused by extremes of anger or fear, emotions that elevate the level of yellow bile, the bitter alkaline secretions in the stomach. When there is too much yellow bile in the system, it causes inflammation in the stomach, intestines, or liver. In the Chinese system of medicine, humors were subclassified into yin and yang, feminine and masculine components, a division that continues to figure largely in Chinese medicine today.

The ancient Chinese principle that food has hot and cold properties, which cause similar physical conditions, also came with the Spanish to the New World. Foods were considered hot or cold in essence rather than in actual temperature, and certain combinations were considered healthy or unhealthy. This "hot and cold" theory is still useful for me today because parts of it make experiential sense. I know that there are certain mixtures of foods that cause physical illness and others that will heal. For example, in my tradition we never serve milk and pork at the same time because eating these two "cold" foods together results in poor digestion or *empacho* (blockage of the intestines). Certain physical conditions are considered hot and cold and should be treated accordingly. As a teenager I was often cautioned, when menstruating, to avoid eating lemons and bananas. I never questioned why; I just didn't eat them. Now I know that this is because menstruation is a "warm" condition, and both of these fruits are "cold" to the system and might cause menstrual cramps. When we shed menstrual blood, there is increased energy in our system, sending our body temperature higher.

Sometimes cold conditions are treated with cold foods. For example, if someone had *susto*, a cold condition, splashing cold water onto the patient's face is a better treatment than warm water because the soul must be shocked back into the body. The result is similar to the scenes from the old movies in which a hysterical person has a glass of ice water thrown into his face, immediately calms down, and says, "Thanks, I needed that."

Certain aspects of the hot and cold theory used in Spanish medicine were adopted by the Native Americans in the New World because they complemented the concept of balance and harmony that the indigenous people practiced. Some ideas relating to the hot and cold theory are still practiced by curanderos in Mexico today.

The Spiritual Theory. The Spanish also believed in an approach to sickness that placed the responsibility for an illness on events that were linked with curses, *mal ojo* (the evil eye), punishment for sins, and magic. In general, illness was considered an effect of a possession by evil spirits, resulting from not following God's laws.

The spiritual type of medicine was what the Spanish promoted throughout the majority of the population of countries that they conquered. The rational-scientific approach was reserved for the elite in power, such as the Spanish governors, prosperous miners, and owners of haciendas.

Even though some modern curanderos, or at least the scholars who write about them, still talk about hexes and *brujería* (black witchcraft), I would like to make it clear that I personally have had little or no experience of it. I don't know any brujos who do the things that many academic papers claim they do. I have never met anyone who collects graveyard dust, mixes it with urine and feces, and concocts evil spells to put on people. As a modern-day curandera, however, what I *do* see are people who come to me because they feel that they have been hexed or cursed, and some of them feel as if the person who cursed them went to a specialist to get help.

There are certain things that I am sure of. I know that when we send negative thoughts to someone, it does harm to him and it comes back on us. I also know, from experience, that there are curanderas who take money from people, sometimes thousands of dollars, and tell their clients that they will do magic to remove a curse; but I think these people are just as evil as the so-called brujos who supposedly cause the curses.

As a curandera, I believe that I have a responsibility to educate and empower people. We may have no control over those who wish us ill, but we do have control over our own souls and spirits. People can die from suggestion, if they get frightened enough, but they can also learn how to have strong souls and spirits and protect themselves. I teach my clients to call upon divine guidance, saints that are meaningful to them, and the protective spirits of their ancestors.

Indigenous Medical Systems and Curanderismo: Children of the Conquest

I believe that one of the reasons curanderismo is so powerful is that it is a medicine that developed, in large part, from the incredible healing that took place from the encounter between Europeans, Indians, Africans, and their offspring. There was a need to develop a medicine that could heal the pain and the immense *susto*, soul loss, that resulted from the cultural destruction, enslavement, and rape that occurred during the Spanish Conquest of the Americas. Is it any wonder that the most important illnesses that curanderismo has developed cures for are *susto* and *envidia* (envy)? These diseases came from internalized oppression and the envy of the power of the oppressor.

As a woman of European, Mayan, Zapotec, and Aztec descent, I am a product of the mixing of races resulting from the Spanish Conquest. The first mestizos, those born from the intermixing of the Spaniards and the Indians, were homeless and had no definite place in society. Many of these children were rejected and discarded when the Spaniards returned to their families in Spain, or found Spanish wives in the New World. Mestizos were agonizing reminders to Indians of the Conquest and the defeat of their culture, religion, and souls. When African slaves were later brought to the New World, they experienced the same suffering and oppression. But somehow we descendants of those outcasts of mixed blood have survived, which is a reflection of how strong our spirits are. We have shared our medicines with one another, as well as our diseases and pain.

Curanderismo is the gift that our ancestors left us. African and indigenous Americans have not healed completely, and we still suffer from the effects of detribalization, soul loss, and envy, but in curanderismo the secrets of our ancient folklore and healing have been preserved and continue to grow.

Gifts of the Aztecs: The "Greatest Medicine"

The advanced medical systems of many Native American tribes, including the Mayans, have contributed greatly to the development of curanderismo, but for now I wish to focus primarily on the culture I have been apprenticed to for the last fourteen years, the Aztec. At the time of the Spanish Conquest, the expression of art, medicine, and culture developed by the Aztecs in the cities of Texcoco and Tenochtitlán was very sophisticated and impressive. The word *Aztec* comes from a Spanish word meaning "people who created technology," and reflects the Conquistadores' wonder at this advanced civilization. This indigenous group refer to themselves as the Mexihka. The Aztec civilization had developed superb architecture, sculptural arts, poetry, pictograph manuscripts, an exact science of time, a complex religion, and a tremendous knowledge of medicine and herbs. Aztec medicine was highly spiritual, and sacred forces were included in all its treatments and diagnosis.

What many people do not realize is that the Aztecs did not disappear after the Spanish Conquest, but continue to live throughout Mexico, concentrated in the central part of the country and in Mexico City. There are hundreds of thousands who still keep their traditions. While I do not know exactly what Aztec medicine and philosophy was like at the time of the Conquest, I do know what my teachers, Andres Segura and Ehekateotl Kuauhtlinxan, have taught me of the medicine that they and their ancestors have preserved. There are several categories of people who are charged with the keeping and the teaching of the medicine and knowledge of the tribe. The first are the **tlamatinime** (possessors of the earth in hand). These are the spiritual wise men and scientists who have firsthand knowledge of the character or nature of things. They function as healers, teachers, philosophers, and spiritual leaders. They conduct soul retrievals by reproducing for their patients their "face and heart," their true identity.

The **teixkitomanitl**. Literally translated as "he who removes the stone from the eye," this person is a doctor similar to an ophthalmologist, a doctor who specializes in treating certain visual defects. The *teixkitomanitl* also attends to spiritual vision, helping his patents to see the errors committed in their relationships with their families and community.

Titzitl (the only one). When another doctor does not know what is causing an illness and cannot cure it, he would send you to a *titzitl*, a healer of great practical experience who will almost always be able to cure the really difficult cases.

Tepahtianikeh (carrier of the medicine stone). This healer is similar to our general practitioners in that he does not have a specialty but attends to the general health of the community.

Tetzkowapanin (one who generates identity). This doctor is a specialist who deals with emotional problems, such as grief over the loss of a loved one. He works with the soul, *(newatl)* and helps you to understand your true identity.

The *tepatiani* is a doctor who specializes in massage. The full name for this method is *apapaxtli tlawayotl maihpahtli*. When this phrase is broken down a beautiful concept emerges. According to my teacher, Ehekateotl, *apapaxtli* means *apapachar*, which in Spanish is a common expression of love, but the word also means "to soften." Tlawayotl means "what is generated from the heart of the people," and *maihpahtli* signifies "the hands that heal." So the complete idea is "to soften what the heart of the people generate with hands that heal." In modern day curanderismo, the *tepatiani* is now referred to as a *sobador* (massage therapist).

My teacher, Ehekateotl Kuauhtlinxan, whose first name means "Essence of the Atmosphere" and whose last name means "The Nest of the Eagle," is a *médico* and instructor of the traditional health system *Wewepahtli* (The Greatest Medicine). Among his people, he is known as the "carrier of the word" for the continuation of the *Tetzkatlipoka* (the gray smoky mirror) tradition. This tradition represents one of the four quadrants of the Aztec altar and is one of the four branches of the culture that, taken all together, describes the philosophy of how human beings should live together in community. The teachings of the gray smoky mirror tradition are passed down through a generational system, from father to son, mother to daughter, and instructor to apprentice. Ehekateotl is in charge of conveying the ceremonies, instruction, and culture of this tradition for future generations.

According to Ehekateotl, *Wewepahtli* combines four great techniques. The first, which is called *matzewallitztli,* means "deserving." Good health is a choice, something that we work to deserve by practicing healthy customs and habits. We must learn how to rest properly and how to provide our bodies with good nutrition. One of the most important concepts of Aztec medicine, and one that I stress with my clients, is taking responsibility for your own health and illness. Ehekateotl tells a story of a man who keeps cutting his hand over and over because he is careless. He can go to the best healers in the world, but his hand will not stay whole if he keeps on neglecting himself. Taking responsibility for your illness, letting go of false belief systems that hurt you, and educating yourself about a healthy lifestyle are important components of wellness that curanderismo inherited from the Aztecs.

The second technique is called *pahtlitztli,* which refers to the management or handling of everything used for medicine, whether these medications be of vegetable, animal, mineral, or gaseous origin. Herbology is included in this category. Aztec healers are wonderful herbalists. They have documented over 300 medicinal herbs and their uses, and Mexican herbs are among the most effective in the world.

The third type of medicine is called *apapaxtli tlawayotl maihpahtli,* which includes physical manipulation, massage, and bodywork.

The fourth category of medicine is known as the *pahwawtztli,* which refers to the instruments of healing, natural tools such as bunches of flowers or the feathers of birds (used in *limpias*), minerals, and tools designed by human beings such as the *tematzkalli*, the sacred sweat lodge.

The Essence of the Four Movements

The system I continue to study with Ehekateotl is called the *nawi ollin teotl*, (the essence of the four movements). The "greatest medicine" is part of the *nawi ollin teotl* system, which is comprised of an ancestral formula that shows the correct proportions used to keep all the organic workings and relationships within the human body in balance, including nutrition, the use of herbs, the proper use of the breath, exercise, and self-evaluation. It also teaches us how we should form proper, balanced relationships with our selves, our partners, our families, our community, and the universe. The *nawi ollin teotl* system is the ancestral formula used by the indigenous pueblos of Mexico to make decisions regarding health, spirit, relationships, nutrition, and everything that has to do with life and the life of the universe.

When the Spaniards recorded the names of the Aztec gods and goddesses Quetzalcoatl, Huitzilopochtli, Coyolxauhqui, and Coatlique in their histories, they were laboring under a very basic misunderstanding. To the Aztecs, who do not believe in "God" in the same sense that we do, these names refer not to all-powerful, omniscient beings but to energies and cosmic forces. To them, the balance and movement of energies, both human and divine, is very sacred, and a good part of their practice of the spiritual hinges around this idea. The universal forces and movements of the cosmos are divided into four quadrants with *Ometeotl*, the sum of all this energy, in the center. Another way to envision these energies is to see them as the philosophical principles underlying the energy of the universe.

The main goal of the Aztecs is to live in harmony with this universe, of which they are a part. They believe that the universe is made up of an immense net of energy channels that meet and combine at different points. If everything is in balance, what they refer to as supreme equilibrium exists.

Just as equilibrium is important for the universal energies, it is also important in the human realm. Through centuries of observation and practice, the Aztecs have come up with mathematical formulas for balancing human, family, community, and spiritual life. This formula is based upon the following proportions: 52 percent, 26 percent, 13 percent, and 9 percent, all of which add up to 100 percent. For example 52 percent of basic human health depends upon proper respiration, 26 percent upon resting and sleeping, 13 percent upon proper hydration, and 9 percent upon proper nutrition. This adds up to 100 percent equilibrium, which makes up basic life because it allows our energy to move in the most efficient way possible.

We can apply these same proportions to all aspects of life. A proper nutritional balance would be made up of 52 percent grains, 26 percent vegetables, 13 percent fruits, and 9 percent protein. To have healthy relationships we would need to put 52 percent of our energy toward our evolving self, 26 percent toward our families, 13 percent toward our community, and 9 percent toward the universe.

If our aim is what the Aztecs refer to as supreme equilibrium, 52 percent of our energy goes toward the maintenance of our own health, the health of our families and our communities, and the health of the universe. If we are not healthy, we cannot generate anything but survival. Twenty-six percent of our energy goes toward the maintenance of our free-dom, because we need to be a free, creative, productive, and solvent people who have an intact culture and traditions. Thirteen percent goes toward acquiring wisdom, which comes from apprenticeship and learning, followed by years of practicing and developing what we have learned. Nine per-cent goes toward the maintenance of our conscience, which allows us, ultimately, to be of service to others.

For healers, taking a vow to be of service challenges us to go through all these steps in order to have the *energy* to be of service. But this ancestral and very wise system is not just for healers, it is for everyone. Wise people need to help other people along the way, to be of service, and to pass on the knowledge that they have gained. This is why my tradition honors our elders and ancestors who have greater experience than we younger people do.

Reclaiming the Past

It has not been easy for me to learn what I have learned about this medicine. Books and scholarly research told me little, and many articles written about the Aztec medical practices at the time of the Spanish Conquest were based on myth and misconception. As I learned about the medicine from my Aztec teachers, I began to see that even the Aztec words themselves, which contain the sounds of nature and the goal of harmony, had been misunderstood or mistranslated.

Many modern researchers of curanderismo portray this medicine as standing still, as if it weren't still continually growing and evolving. They dismiss the medicine as prescientific medical quackery. One researcher baldly stated that curanderismo is used only to treat certain folk disorders that are "unique to Mexican Americans, and do not affect Anglo Americans." Everyone has a soul and a spirit, and everyone is susceptible to envy, rage, and loss of identity! Other investigators claim that curanderismo is still being used only because it is cheaper than Western medicine and poor Mexican Americans cannot afford better care. In my practice I treat people of all ethnic backgrounds, professionals and blue-collar workers, the rich, the middle class, and the poor.

The picture of curanderismo that I am presenting in this book is much wider, broader, and richer than any of the definitions I have found on the shelves of libraries. Many of the old wisdom keepers died without passing on what they knew because my generation and my parents' generation were being pressured to assimilate, to turn our backs on the old beliefs. I have sought out many of those old wise ones who are still living, but they have not always been able to explain to me *why* they do what they do. Most of the time they tell me that they heal that way because their grandmother did. For example, I often ask curanderas why they use an egg when they do *limpias*. I have never yet received a satisfactory answer. For that reason, I resisted using the egg for many years. When I finally decided to try this tool, I was amazed at what I discovered. For the last eleven years I have done an average of two or three *limpias* a day, four or five days a week. If you do the math, that adds up to literally thousands of *limpias*. During that time, I have been astonished at how rubbing an egg over someone's body has helped me to read their energy. This tool has become a doorway that helps me to read people's souls.

For many years people referred to folk medicine as "alternative," eventually graduating to the term "complementary." I am writing this book because I believe that the time has come for us to take a serious look at how traditional medicine not only complements modern mainstream medicine but surpasses it in many ways. As a psychiatric nurse with a master's degree and a curandera of twenty-three years, I feel that I am a woman of two worlds—both the traditional and the modern. From this standpoint, I would like to help the reader to examine the strengths and weaknesses of both. In a modern HMO the patient must wait two months for an appointment, and then only gets to see the doctor for fifteen minutes. This kind of health care simply cannot compare with the loving care one receives from a holistic practitioner or a curandera who welcomes your tears, does not put time limits on how long you can speak, touches your body in a loving and sacred way, and creates personalized ceremonies to strengthen your spirit and help you to find the lost parts of your soul.

Many people today are frustrated with Western medicine because they know that it lacks heart. What I am offering in this book is another approach, one that teaches that every man and woman alive already possesses the "greatest medicine" within them. No one can really cure another human being. True healing is always a *cocreation* between client and healer, as the dozens of stories of men and women told in this book show. A medical system that encourages people not to ask questions and to accept blindly the treatments and prescriptions of a doctor, and teaches nothing about preventative measures, nutrition, or how to maintain emotional health is lacking in the most basic tenets of health *care.*

Curanderismo teaches that it is not enough to diagnose a physical problem, as so many modern medical doctors do, without also looking at what is going on in the heart and soul of the patient. Each illness is a story, and only the patient can tell that story. I have seen many cases where sicknesses have been cured using modern methods, but a few months later, the illness comes back again because the problem in the *soul* has never been dealt with. Only a medicine that deals with the whole being can effectively create a whole cure.

True healing must go deep and take time to be permanent. The soul will always find ways to manifest its hurts, regardless of what is cured. Most important, true healing can only be effective if it has some kind of spiritual basis. In my work, I do not care what spiritual system my clients cherish, only that they know how to call upon divine energy to help them in their healing. We are all spiritual beings, and we cannot experience true wellness if we do not fully acknowledge that.

The history of how allopathic medicine became the only official medicine in the U.S. is a long story that is beyond the scope of this book. Some of the Europeans who first immigrated to this country came fleeing the Spanish Inquisition when thousands of traditional healers were sent to the torturer's dungeon or put to the torch. Perhaps these immigrants internalized their fear and distrust of folk medicine when they came to this country. Much knowledge was lost during those years, and only recently have people begun to reclaim it. I have certainly had to sift through the bones of my own ancestors to unearth my own tradition. It is my hope that this book will inspire others to go back to their own roots and discover the medicine of their ancestors.

I did not invent curanderismo. I am only the vehicle for its transmission. I do not conquer the nature of my patients, I release it. True medicine is not just passively accepting an herbal tea or a pill from a practitioner who has no knowledge of natural living. There is a medicine that can be triggered from within each and every one of us and we all have the potential to heal ourselves and our global family. Curanderismo is not just a medical practice but a whole culture of health. It is a culture that seeks equilibrium between the self and nature by engaging the cosmos, by learning to honor natural laws, customs, traditions, energetic systems, and social systems, as well as our personal biological system. Illness is not seen as an individual problem. It is viewed as an imbalance in which one individual becomes the focus of the healing process that in the end will purify and balance all of the systems and community or family members involved. In this book, it is my wish to honor the elders who kept this knowledge alive despite discrimination, persecution, and even death.

To be responsible for one's health should be in the conscience of every person so that we can stop being beggars of those whom we believe possess greater knowledge. Through reading the stories of everyday people presented in this book, I hope readers will be inspired to possess the "greatest medicine" for themselves, their family, and all living things in our global community.

E.A. and J.P.

Chapter One

Curanderismo
Health Care for the Body and *Soul*

Curanderismo treats problems that are recognized as illnesses in Western medicine, as well as many that aren't. I have treated people with eating disorders, diabetes, heart problems, cancer, chronic back problems, hypertension, and just about anything that a medical doctor treats. I have also worked with people who were struggling with shyness, self-consciousness, a broken heart, bad luck, a wish for greater prosperity, nightmares, envy, loneliness, rage, anxiety, family

41

problems, marriage problems, sexual problems, infertility, how to find a partner, or how to leave a partner.

Some clients come to me saying that they have no ambition and don't know how to find the energy to get ahead in their careers. Others come because they are collapsing under the stress of too much ambition. Patients have sat in my treatment room and told me that they have lost faith in life and need a cure for hopelessness. Others come with health problems that they feel are not being adequately treated by their medical doctors. By coming to a curandera, they are acknowledging that medical science can take them only so far, and that some diseases will only heal when the wounds of the heart and soul have been healed as well.

More and more people today are using the services of both a medical doctor *and* a curandera. I see people in my treatment room diagnosed with gastrointestinal disorders, diabetes, hypertension, arthritis, chronic fatigue syndrome, and migraine headaches, among other illnesses. Some of them come to see me because they would like to try a more holistic approach in their treatment. Some feel uncomfortable with the side-effects of the medication they are taking and want to know if there are alternative therapies, such as herbs. Many do not really understand their illness and complain that their doctor does not take enough time to educate them. As a trained nurse and curandera, I explain the nature of their problem and how it is manifesting in their individual physiology. I refer them to articles, books, and Internet Web pages that talk about their disease, and tell them what their alternatives are for treatment.

I occasionally see clients who are in denial about their illness, and hope that a curandera will give them a more acceptable diagnosis. Some clients want to believe that the strange behaviors and thoughts that they or their loved ones are producing are the result of a curse. I have seen many people diagnosed with the chemical imbalance of schizophrenia who are frankly psychotic but want to believe that they are sick because someone has put a hex on them. I have assisted many of these individuals by helping them accept their illness and find creative ways to live their lives.

It is always a challenge and a source of great satisfaction for me to search for ways to meet the physical, emotional, and spiritual needs of all of these people. Not everyone is willing to dedicate himself to the time, education, and hard work that it takes to become a whole, healthy person, but I have witnessed the transformation of hundreds of clients who came to me with very serious emotional and physical diseases. Curanderos love to see miracles happen—but we and our clients have to work hard for our miracles, cocreating wellness together.

"Folk" Diseases

To really understand curanderismo, it is necessary to look at the way that curanderos categorize disease. Any book or academic study of curanderismo always lists certain "classic" illnesses, so we will take a look at all of them here. In the last few decades, however, curanderismo has gone through some changes. Like any form of health care, it has not stood still in the modern world. Some conditions, such as *susto* (soul loss), envy, and *bilis* (rage) are still treated often by curanderos. Other disciplines, such as the work of the *partera* (the midwife) are seldom used in the U.S. since the advent of the widespread use of modern hospitals and birthing centers. *Parteras* still catch babies and attend to the pre- and postnatal care of women in rural Mexico and Guatemala, but no longer in the U.S. border towns. What we can learn from the few vanishing specialties of curanderismo, however, is their holistic wisdom about the care of the whole person, body and soul.

Curanderos treat physical diseases, such as *bilis, empacho,* and *mal aire*; mental diseases such as *envidia, mal puesto, mal ojo,* and *mal suerte;* and spiritual diseases such as *susto* and *espanto.* Let's take a look at each of these categories.

I. Physical Diseases

Bilis (rage) is caused by the excess secretion of bile that floods the system when a person is suffering from chronic rage. This is certainly an illness that many people in modern society suffer from, and Western culture is rife with terms that describe it, such as "rage-aholic." This condition causes digestive problems and toxicity to the body, especially the liver, stomach, and intestines. A curandero cures *bilis* by relaxing the patient with massage, and prescribing soothing herbal teas and baths. In curanderismo, it is especially important that the patient be educated about the dangers of repressing anger and fear, and how to express anger in a healthy manner. Rage is destructive not only to a patient but to the rest of his or her family. If a parent is rageful, the children and partner can become sick with *susto*, soul loss. Rage can also lead to domestic violence and child abuse.

When I was a child, my mother suffered from terrible attacks of *bilis*. Terrified of her anger, I used to hide on the back porch until it subsided. When my father drank, my mother would go into rages and they would have violent fights. I remember how frightening it was for my sisters and me to be yanked from our beds at night by my mother during one of these fights. We would have to go to a neighbor's house until the battle subsided. I hated my father's drinking and my mother's rage, and I can personally attest to their destructive effects upon a family.

Later, when I was myself a mother and found myself reacting in rage to my own children, I would remember that scared little child that I'd been who hid under the house until her mother's *bilis* subsided. This memory would motivate me to work on my own *bilis*. I remember going into the bathroom and counting to ten when my son, Adrian, who was born with brain damage and mental retardation, was especially hard to handle. He used rage to get his needs met, and when he was upset, he would cry for long periods of time. I could not calm him, and it was difficult to manage the rage within me, born out of my frustration and feelings of inadequacy. Finally I sought the help of a healer who utilized a method that he called rage reduction. He showed me a technique for holding my son that facilitated a positive bonding experience that reduced the *bilis* in both of us. My work with this healer not only improved my relationship with my son but with the rest of my children as well. I incorporated this method into my own practice and have been using it successfully ever since. Adrian is now twenty-seven and we have a close and loving relationship. A few months ago he left home and now holds a full-time job and lives independently with four other young men.

Empacho refers to a blockage of the stomach or the digestive tract. It can come from overeating, food allergies, lactose intolerance, eating when not hungry, or eating hard-to-digest foods. Metaphorically, curanderos also use this term to describe any kind of blocks to the emotional or energy body.

When I was a child, I often suffered from *empacho.* My mother warned me about eating uncooked tortilla dough but, since kids are famous for testing, I sneaked some anyway. Sure enough, I got sick with *empacho.* I also hated being forced to eat Cream of Wheat every morning. I could not leave the table until I had finished it. This was torture for me and, on several occasions, I ended up with *empacho* and vomited the cereal all over the place, which enraged my mom. My little stomach knew that foods we are forced to eat never sit well with us.

One time when an Anglo girlfriend was making a cake and licked the bowl clean with the spatula, I was shocked. "Aren't you afraid of getting *empacho?*" I asked her. She did not know what I was talking about, and I was surprised that she had been eating uncooked dough since she was a kid and had never gotten a stomachache.

The power of suggestion may be what influences some individuals to contract *empacho,* but almost everybody has had this condition at one time or another. *Empacho* can cause gas, stomach cramps, diarrhea, constipation, loss of appetite, and vomiting. The *sobadora* (massage therapist) knows how to massage the stomach and the lower back to unblock the *empacho,* and will prescribe different herbal teas, such as *yerba buena* (peppermint) and *manzanilla* (chamomile) to soothe the digestive tract. Avoiding *empacho* involves paying attention to how our bodies react to the things we eat, especially sugar, white flour, fat, spicy foods, chocolate, and coffee. Sometimes the foods that our minds love are not very well tolerated by our bodies.

Codependent people can develop *empacho* of the heart from "loving too much." Women are especially susceptible to this form of *empacho*. When we lose ourselves in another person, an energy block develops that prevents us from growing emotionally. We can also get *empacho* from being around someone else's toxic energy. A common saying is *"Me tiene em-pachado"* ("He has me *empachado*," meaning "blocked"). Or a person can have *empacho* of the soul. For example, I had been wanting to write a book on curanderismo for years, but had not had the time nor the opportunity. My mind was so filled with information that needed to come out that I was suffering from a spiritual and emotional *empacho* that was blocking the energy in my soul. When a person is filled with ideas that she needs to express, or something that she needs to create, she must find an outlet for this energy or *empacho* may result.

Mal Aire (bad air) is a disease that manifests with cold symptoms, earaches, or facial paralysis, and is often caused by prolonged exposure to the night air. Children are especially susceptible to *mal aire,* and one of the traditional ways to avoid this illness is to make sure that very young children are swaddled tightly in blankets before taking them out at night. The customs that protect children from *mal aire* go all the way back to before the time of the Spanish Conquest in Mexico and reflect the fact that the indigenous tribes, including the Aztecs, knew that chilling the body made it more vulnerable to disease. These tribes were also aware that diseases were caused by airborne bacteria, even though they called these

tiny organisms by different names. My Aztec teacher, Ehekateotl, told me, "The Aztecs knew that tiny particles in the air
could make people sick. They did not understand about mi-
crobes so they called these particles spirits. These particles
would go through changes and enter the body, making people
sick, paralyzing the face, or causing colds. They would fly
around the person and penetrate the body. This was over four
hundred seventy-five years ago." Ehe explained to me how,
even today, scholars misunderstand what the Aztecs at the
time of the Conquest were really talking about when they
translate the terms they used, and still use, for their medicine.
"We approached illness holistically, and we did have our
words, our language, to explain illness. We used our language
and it has been translated inaccurately. Modern people fail to
comprehend this." For example, when Indian women sang
lullabyes to the Spanish children they cared for, singing,
"Coco, coco," the Spaniards completely misunderstood. *"Coco"*
means "the boogie man" in Spanish, while in Nahuatl it simply means "go to sleep." So, while the Indian women were
singing, "Sleep so that you can rest and not get sick," the
Spaniards thought they were saying, "The boogie man is
going to get you if you don't sleep." We have to be careful
when we translate from one language to the next because
much can be lost in the process. The Aztec language is
much more right-brain than Spanish or English, much more
metaphorical.

One of the most important things that Ehekateotl told me
about the practice of swaddling a child with blankets to protect it from *mal aire* was that this was originally more of a
metaphor for protection than a health rule that could not be
broken. Wrapping the child in blankets was seen as a way of

swaddling it with love and protection. I wish someone had told me this when I was a young woman, always trying to do the right thing for my children according to the traditions I had been raised with. When I was seventeen, I gave birth to my first child, Jamie. Nine months later, we moved to West Berlin to join my husband who was stationed there in the air force. My husband had to work long shifts, so I was on my own quite a bit.

One day I noticed that Jamie had a high fever. I gave him baby aspirin, but it didn't seem to have any effect. He didn't want to wake up from his nap, and every time I touched him, he felt hotter and hotter. I felt so young, alone, and powerless. We lived off base and I did not speak German. I kept trying to reach my husband to ask for help, but when Jamie woke up and started having a convulsion, I couldn't wait any longer. I frantically phoned the army hospital and was told to bring my son to the emergency room. I called a taxi, wrapped my baby up with a blanket, covering his face as my mother had taught me to do to prevent *mal aire.*

When I arrived at the hospital, the doctor took one look at my swaddled son, and began to yell at me, "Your son is burning up with fever. He just had a fever convulsion and needs to cool down. Are you trying to kill him? What is the matter with you people?" (meaning Mexican Americans). Completely humiliated, I felt as if I were a horrible mother. I hated my culture for almost killing my son, and I felt shame for believing in *mal aire,* in bad spirits that could harm a child when he was taken outside and exposed to the air. It was not the old belief about swaddling the child that was wrong, however. It was my misunderstanding of its real purpose.

Later, when I was Director of Maternal/Child Nursing at

R. E. Thomason General Hospital in El Paso, Texas, I started a teaching program for mothers and the nursing personnel. I explained to them the real meaning of *mal aire,* and the importance of cooling a child down with tepid water when he has a fever. I let them know that it is better to dress a child lightly until the fever goes down. I never want a mother to suffer the shame and guilt I felt when that doctor insulted me, or to make her child's illness worse by practicing incorrect beliefs about *mal aire.* I told my classes, just as I tell my clients who are mothers now, "We swaddle our children with love and protective intent."

II. Mental Diseases

The term "mental illness" means something different to a curandero than it does to a modern medical doctor, because curanderismo never treats the mind in isolation from a person's body, emotions, soul, and spirit. As a psychiatric nurse who has worked with the mentally ill for many years, I know from experience that this is exactly the kind of treatment that is missing in our mental institutions. Curanderos do treat medically diagnosed mental illnesses, but they always look at the patient's entire being. As a curandera, I often work with the mentally ill, helping them find a way to cope with their medications and become more stable emotionally. I educate their families on what to expect from these illnesses, and how to act and respond in ways that make life easier on everyone.

Mental illnesses can be the result of either deep traumas or a chemical imbalance due to genetic factors. But a person does not have to succumb to his illness. He does not have to fall into despair and feel that his life is over. If a diabetic did not take his medication and follow his diet and exercise regime, he would get worse. The same is true of the mentally ill. Unfortunately many patients do not like the side effects of their psychotropic drugs and instead choose to suffer the hallucinations and paranoia that can occur when they do not take the drugs.

My Aztec teacher, Ehekateotl, believes that if we can learn to generate enough energy by keeping our bodies healthy, we will also have the energy to keep our emotions and our minds as healthy as possible. If we can retain a strong spirit and soul, we can learn to live in greater harmony and balance with our afflictions, whatever they may be. I have learned much from the schizophrenics, manic, and depressed individuals with whom I work. Many of them have big hearts, strong bodies, and a strong spirit and soul. They respond well to the spiritual cleansings and soul retrievals I do with them, and to the education I give them. But most of all, they respond to compassion.

III. Emotional Diseases

Envídia (envy) affects a person in one of two distinct ways. The first way concerns the envious individual, the person who is sick in her soul. The second concerns the *envied* individual, the person who is receiving energy that is not hers. When someone is the object of envy, she gets sick in her *tonal* (spirit). How does one receive envious energy? We can all think of times when someone envied us, and how painful that was — times when someone hated us because we had a new job, a master's degree, a loving relationship, or a new car. Envy is an energy that is contrary to love, and when someone feels that emotion, she can transmit it by her presence without saying anything. Even people we love, friends and family members, can harm us without meaning to.

Envy is the twist in the heart that we feel in the presence of someone else's good fortune. This feeling always offers us a choice, however, because it shows us the things that our souls really long for. We can choose to focus on feelings of impotence because someone else has what we do not have, allowing envy to eat away at our hearts until it has become a destructive, debilitating force in our lives, or we can do the work that needs to be done in order to achieve what the object of our envy has achieved. Sometimes that means going back to school, or working hard for a promotion at work, or leaving a bad relationship and seeking a healthier one. When we use envy as a mirror, we can achieve our goals at work, school, and in our personal life faster.

Mal Puesto (a hex or curse). Many people in the part of the world where I live believe that *mal puesto* is a result of the "black magic" kind of witchcraft. I have never met a practitioner of black magic, but I do believe that evil people exist who intentionally attempt to harm others out of envy, revenge, or greed. I also know that there are individuals who profit from people's cultural beliefs in *mal puesto* because I have treated hundreds of patients who have paid so-called curanderas large sums of money to remove a hex or curse from them.

Charlatans and impersonators of curanderismo have learned how to profit from people's fears. Many of these people claim that they can divine the source of a hex using Tarot cards, trance states, aura readings, *limpias*, astrology, spiritualism, fortune telling, palm readings, or psychic readings. Since they use many of the same tools that competent curanderas use, it is sometimes difficult to distinguish a quack from an authentic healer. These imposters are often astute and unethical people who can "read" body language, making them appear to be psychic. Their knowledge of human behavior is profound, and gullible patients are seduced into trusting them. Their business flourishes because there are always people who do not want to take responsibility for what is happening in their lives, but want instead to find an outside cause on which to blame their misfortune.

Recently, I saw an elder named Anna who had given a "curandero" her life savings—ten thousand dollars—to take away a hex. I was deeply saddened by her story. Her thirty-six-year-old daughter had been diagnosed as having paranoid schizophrenia but was refusing to take her medication. Anna's daughter was neglecting her small children and was not eating because she believed that her food was poisoned. Anna, who was desperate and could not handle her small grandchildren, had heard about a woman who could cure mental illness. This so-called curandera read the Tarot and told Anna that her daughter had been bewitched by her own father. She could take away the curse, the curandera said, but she had to go to Mexico and buy the necessary materials for the cure. Since it would be a very difficult cure, the materials were very expensive.

My poor client never participated in the "curing ceremony," but did take her savings from the bank and pay the imposter without telling her husband. The curandera's claim that her husband had cursed his own daughter upset and confused Anna deeply, and she even thought of ending their forty-five-year marriage.

When the promised cure did not take effect and her daughter did not get better, Anna brought her daughter to see me. It was obvious to me that her daughter had a chronic condition and needed to take her medication. Not taking her medicine was what was causing her to become violent with her children.

Anna will never recover her life savings, but she was able to accept her daughter's illness. I did a *plática* and a *limpia* with her daughter, and explained why I did not support her belief that she was cursed. I also helped the daughter to accept her illness and to explore all of her alternatives for treatment. She decided she was willing to take her medication and is now doing better. Anna's relationship with both her daughter and her husband has improved and she has learned a valuable lesson about not trusting healers who demand huge sums of money for their services.

I see many individuals who believe they have been cursed, but, in reality, are suffering from a form of mental illness. In such cases, my training as a psychiatric nurse and my many years of experience on hospital psychiatric wards have stood me in good stead. While I am not able to cure people suffering from diseases such as paranoid schizophrenia, I can certainly help them to live happier lives. For example, paranoid schizophrenics need to be taught to talk about their fears. If someone says, "Good morning" to them in a way that they perceive is wrong, they can become upset and fearful. I teach them how to express these fears by, perhaps, asking, "Are you mad at me this morning?" It is reassuring for them to hear, "No, I just have a lot on my mind today and I am a bit preoccupied." I also refer people with psychiatric illnesses to support groups, encourage them not to give in to the desire to isolate themselves from others, and refer them to medical doctors if I think they would benefit from medication or a period of hospitalization. Since mental and emotional illnesses are always a family issue, I also educate the patient's family about how they can help.

Often I help people release the shame that surrounds mental illness and the need to take psychotropic drugs by saying things to them such as "schizophrenia is a genetic disease. You haven't done anything wrong, it's not your fault." Or, "Taking medications is nothing to be ashamed of. A lot of people have to take medications for long periods of time. Diabetics have to take insulin every day." Releasing that shame is an important part of learning to live with mental illness.

Most important, I give such individuals and their families the spiritual strength they need to accept the parameters of the illness. When we develop spiritual strength, we can open new doors.

I have had personal experience with charlatans who are expert at nurturing fear and separating people from their life savings. A few years ago I heard that there was a powerful curandera practicing in Juárez, Mexico. My sister Irma and I decided to check her out, and I presented the woman with a real problem that I was having.

The curandera began by giving me a penetrating look, and saying, "Oh, so you are a healer!" I was impressed and she had my attention. She looked at the family pictures she had asked me to bring and made a few general statements that had some truth in them. Then she took me to another room and gave me a *limpia* with an egg. When she was finished, she handed the egg to her assistant who was standing behind me. The assistant dropped the egg into a glass of water and handed the glass to the curandera. There was a small dead lizard in the glass with the egg and the curandera got a shocked look on her face. I have done thousands of *limpias* with eggs and have never seen anything other than the egg in the glass. Realizing that I was being set up, I immediately lost my confidence in the healer.

Here it comes, I thought, the hook. "Many generations back, an envious and revengeful person put a hex on your family," the curandera told me. "Your family has had illness and bad luck ever since because this person cursed your family for many generations. Your family will never be happy unless this curse is removed."

"How much will the cure cost?" I said, trying to pretend innocence.

"Four thousand dollars," was her reply. Irma and I thanked her and told her we would be in touch with her. "Do not wait too long," she warned. We went to Irma's house and gave each other a *limpia* to take away the bad energy from this charlatan.

Many reputable curanderas will not treat *mal puesto* because of the fear that they will be called *brujas* (witches). I do treat *mal puesto*, but I make it very clear that I do not believe in curses.

It is not just people from my cultural tradition who come to see me because they believe they have been hexed. On occasion, even professional people such as doctors or lawyers have come into my treatment room, stuttering and beating around the bush. "Uh, do you think there is really such a thing as . . . I mean, have you ever seen people who are . . . I mean, do you think that people can be, uh, cursed?" In such cases, I do not encourage the belief, but help these people to understand what is really happening in their lives and to take responsibility for their problems. When our lives feel out of control, when we are having a run of bad luck, it is easy to believe that someone has put a hex on us. In such cases, it is important for us to examine our relationships, our attitudes, and our emotional and spiritual health.

One woman came to me complaining that her twenty-two-year-old son was cursed because he had flunked school and could not keep a job. When he was at home, he was listless and slept during the day. The mother told me that she suspected his ex-girlfriend had put a curse on him. When I did a *plática* with the son, I found out that he was getting drunk and stoned every night until three in the morning, and was too tired to do anything else. He was cursing himself.

When I treat people, I find it important to educate them about what they consider to be witchcraft. I find it important to empower clients and to guide them into balance and harmony. Many of our misfortunes are the result of our own actions or the ups and downs of everyday life. Our cars break down, a careless driver follows too closely and causes an accident, our children have their problems, and we forget to pay our bills. We eat the wrong foods and drink too much alcohol, work too hard and do not get enough rest. We try to keep up with our neighbors and get envious about their possessions. We have bad thoughts about people and become consumed with revenge. We want to get even with our ex-spouse and find ourselves wishing that he would fail, or get ill, ugly, and fat. We feel lonely and desperate because we are not in a relationship.

I always tell my clients, "Take responsibility for your health and the health of your family. Get out of denial and do something about your unhealthy habits. You are the architect of your life. Don't give your power away. God is much more powerful than any person or 'witch.' God is not punishing you. Put your energy into the development of your soul and spirit. If your spirit is healthy, no harm can penetrate to your soul."

Mal Ojo (or ***mal ∂e ojo***) is one of the most misunderstood diseases in curanderismo. Academic researchers who write articles about curanderismo, or individuals who write books to help health-care workers understand how to give better care to "ethnic minorities," often list folk diseases in simple cultural catalogs that are superficial and erroneous. For example, *mal ojo* has been translated from Spanish into English as "the evil eye." A more accurate translation would be "illness caused by staring," since the word *mal* means "illness," not "evil," in this case. The myth that there is something bad or supernatural connected with *mal ojo* makes people uncomfortable with the term. Human beings fear the supernatural and dualize its energies as either evil or divine. For myself, I do not believe in placing the supernatural outside of ourselves or, for that matter, outside of the natural. We know very little about our potential as human beings. To me, the supernatural represents the animal impulses within all of us, such as sexuality, combined with the unconscious, the unknown, the superhuman, *and* the divine, the God within us.

We have all heard stories of people doing superhuman deeds in times of crisis, and we know that human beings are also capable of great evil. There is nothing "unnatural" in the supernatural.

Some researchers into curanderismo interpret their findings regarding this medicine according to their own theoretical biases, not based on the diverse and holistic ways in which the Chicano culture views illness and wellness. For example, one researcher described *mal ojo* as follows: "The 'evil eye' is an illness to which all children and adults with 'light blood' are susceptible. The blood is believed to be heated by electricity in a stronger person's vision who looks at the afflicted admiringly or covetously but does not touch him. The 'heating' of the blood produces the most often reported symptoms of *ojo*, fever and vomiting."

If I were a nurse or doctor reading this scientific journal, I would wonder about the culture that believes such nonsense. *Mal ojo* is a universal malady that has been identified in cultures all over the world. People's awareness of it is expressed in all kinds of charms and amulets that they use symbolically to protect themselves and their young children from unwanted energies. Some charms are reflective and bounce these energies back to the sender, for example the blue beads used as protective charms in the eastern Mediterranean area. Others are made to look like the eyes of animals with exotic eyes. In the Hispanic culture, charms called *ojo de venado* (deer's eye) are still popular. In Italy, parents place a small talisman, a *figa*, around the necks of infants, to protect them from unwanted attention, and Jewish children and adults wear the *hamesh*, a charm resembling the five fingers of a hand. Women in India draw black lines around their eyes, to protect not only themselves but others from energy that does not belong to them.

In Hispanic cultures, *mal ojo* is the name for the illness that results when too much attention is paid to a very young baby or child. Just ask any mother what happens when she takes an infant to a social function where many well-meaning people stare at it, admire it, and fuss over it. That baby will become distressed and restless, go home cranky, will have trouble sleeping, and might even vomit or run a temperature. This reaction in children is not cultural but universal.

There is an energetic aspect to *mal ojo* that is similar to the energetic exchange that occurs when one person envies another. Babies can *feel* it when a person is staring at them for too long, paying them unwanted attention, pawing them, or overstimulating them. Adults have much more intense and integrated energy fields than does a tiny infant or small child who is new to this world. So in my culture when a person stares at a child or a baby for too long, it is considered common courtesy to touch the child and break the intrusive bond, thus preventing *mal ojo*. We do not stare at beautiful children out of a desire to hurt them. All human beings admire beauty and have a desire to touch and capture that beauty.

My Aztec friend Tzenwaxolokuauhtli, whom his friends call Tzen for short, told me that when he comes to the U.S., he has to be careful about touching a child he is looking at. To him this is both polite and natural, but he is aware that to parents who do not share his cultural values, it might seem offensive or intrusive for a stranger to touch their child. Tzen explained to me that touching a child that we admire changes the vibration that we are sending to that child. "Our eyes are always sending energy to what we are gazing at." The gaze of an adult has a vibration that is not harmonized to that of a child because the child is not capable of meeting the gaze at the same frequency. "When we touch a child, we sense that child's energy, we observe the beauty of that child, and the desire we have to touch the beauty of the child is met." Tzen also says that it is better to touch a child with our left hand because the left hand gives energy, and the right hand removes energy. The left hand is also closer to the heart, so we use that hand to touch with love.

I do not treat many children with this illness, but when I do, I want to be useful. If a parent believes that his or her child is suffering from *mal de ojo,* I know the classical treatment, but I am also on the lookout for a more serious illness. If I find that the child is suffering from some sort of physical disease, I refer him or her to a medical doctor. Many parents already know how to prevent and treat this *mal ojo* by rubbing an egg over their child as prayers are said, or putting a charm or amulet on them. *Mal de ojo* is a short-term illness, which responds well to treatment.

Mala Suerte (bad luck) is seen as an emotional illness because curanderismo believes that the energies and expectations that we put into life have a direct effect on what happens to us. Once we become entangled in low self-esteem, worry, and feelings of helplessness, we can become enmeshed in a vicious cycle of bad luck.

A client of mine named Eva was involved in an automobile accident several months ago in which a driver ran a red light and hit her car on the driver's side. She suffered a broken leg and was out of work for three weeks. Since she had just started a new job and had no sick leave, she was worried about how she was going to pay her bills. One month later she came home one evening and found that her house had been burglarized. The robbers took her television, her VCR, and her gold jewelry. She did not have homeowner's insurance. This made her worry even more, and she began to have trouble sleeping. When she did sleep, she often awoke with nightmares of people chasing her and wanting to hurt her. Because she could not sleep, she became depressed, listless, and irritable, and broke up with her boyfriend. Feeling more depressed than ever, she started to drink heavily. When she went to her doctor to get help, he prescribed an antidepressant, which made her sleepy all day.

When Eva came to see me, she was in a desperate situation. She wanted to know what she had done to deserve such bad luck. I gave her a series of three *limpias* in which she released the energy that did not belong to her, the energy of fear, worry, and distress that she had been carrying around with her since her accident. Some people would call this energy negative, but I simply call it "energy that doesn't belong to us." We most often take on energies that don't belong to us when we are ill, or in a vulnerable place. Eva's broken leg was an accident, and we cannot prevent accidents. Her worry about paying her bills was natural, but, as we all know, worrying does not pay the bills. The other driver's insurance company would have paid Eva's lost wages, but she was too distracted to investigate her options. Since she was distracted, she forgot to lock her house and left it open for the thieves.

In reality, Eva was suffering from a combination of *susto* and bad luck. The car accident and the vandalizing of her house were frightening events that created a soul loss. This state creates an aura that is susceptible to other misfortunes. Eva felt anxious, tense, and angry, so she took those feelings out on her boyfriend, her only emotional support. She was also lonely, so she medicated herself with alcohol. We all know that this only makes matters worse. The magic pill that the doctor gave her did not help; it made her feel worse.

The *limpias* and *pláticas* that I gave Eva changed the vibration of her energy body and her aura, and she began to feel like herself again. She released her "bad luck" and also made important changes in her life. She developed awareness and self-empowerment, and stopped the vicious cycle of bad luck by going right to the source of her problems. She stopped drinking, made up with her boyfriend, received a settlement from the insurance company to pay her bills, and went back to work. Her emotions became balanced and she learned an important lesson that will carry her through her next experience with bad luck.

I think it is good that Eva was aware of the value of curanderismo, and I hope that there will always be curanderos around to treat "bad luck." When we interpret events around us as bad luck, we create a certain vibration around us. Our environment mirrors this energy vibration back to us, and the bad luck takes on a life of its own. There is nothing mystical about this. It's something that anyone can relate to, if they think back on their own experiences with so-called bad luck.

IV. Spiritual (*Tonal*) Diseases

Susto (soul loss). Curanderismo teaches that humans are physical, emotional, mental, and spiritual beings. When all aspects of a person are in harmony with the inner self and the universe, the soul is intact. The spiritual self, the aura that surrounds us, is the most vulnerable to trauma. By our diet, habits, and attitudes, we create an aura that is strong, or weak and full of holes.

If we experience a frightening or traumatic event, this can result in soul loss, a state in which we do not feel fully present or as if we are really ourselves. We experience a feeling that "something is missing" because our spirit, the energetic aura that surrounds us, has been violated. It can either heal quickly or stay injured for a long time, depending on what we do to seek help or help ourselves.

According to Aztec beliefs, in order to have an intact soul, 52 percent of our energy needs to go toward maintaining our physical bodies. This percentage is considered "indispensable" for basic life. If our bodies are healthy, then we have the energy to feel all of our emotions and manage them in a healthy way. Twenty-six percent of our energy needs to be directed toward feeling the full range of our emotions, and managing them in a balanced way. We call this category "necessary." The 13 percent of our energy that we need to maintain the health of our minds is called "desirable," which leads to the 9 percent of our energy that is sufficient to maintain our spirits, which is called "excellent." When the numbers add up to 100 percent in this way, we have a healthy soul, based on a healthy body, mind, emotions, and spirit.

We can't avoid having traumas in our lives, but the way that we recover from shocks and misfortunes has everything to do with how we are able to maintain the health of our soul. Let us look at the recovery process of two women who were raped, one who had a strong, well-protected soul, and one who did not.

Alicia is a thirty-year-old woman who was lucky enough to be healthy physically, mentally, emotionally, and spiritually. One night, she was awakened by a man who broke into her home, tied her up, and raped her. When she came to me for treatment, she was suffering from *susto*. Not only was she traumatized, in shock, sad, angry, and horribly violated, but her spiritual aura had been violated. Everything that she believed in previous to the rape had been shaken and she was in a state of emotional and spiritual paralysis.

Before Alicia could move forward, she needed to reevaluate her life and habits totally. She needed counseling, a trip to a medical doctor for a complete physical, and treatments for soul loss. It might even have been necessary for her to move to a safer side of town for her own peace of mind. But because Alicia had a good sense of her soul (her physical, emotional, mental, and spiritual self) before the rape, the true core of who she is will heal and become intact again. She will be different, because a rape is a great violation of the soul, but she will emerge whole. Her soul will be able to regenerate.

Now let us look at another client named Vicky. Vicky is also thirty years old, but she was a victim of incest when she was five, something that she has never told anyone about. She had frequent kidney infections; her diet consisted of a high fat and sugar intake; and she frequently skipped meals. Her blood pressure was high and she did not have the energy to exercise, which fed her poor body image. Vicky's mind seesawed between extremes of emotions. Some days she hated herself, and at other times she felt superior to other people and isolated herself. She did not have a strong spiritual base and felt that God was punishing her for being "bad." In other words, most of her energy went toward the maintenance of her sick body, and there was very little energy left over for keeping her mind and emotions balanced, much less her spirit.

After she was raped as an adult, Vicky also suffered from soul loss, but her spiritual aura was already deeply trauma- tized—and not just from the present-day rape. Her energetic body had gone through many assaults: her childhood incest and her poor physical health, which had affected her emo- tions, her mind, and her spirit. When Vicky and I began her treatment, the *very last thing* I planned to do with her was a soul retrieval. First I needed to guide her into healing and strengthening all parts of herself. She desperately needed to rebuild the foundation of her being and build up her energy to help her get in touch with her soul—her essence, who she really is. Vicky did not know who she was before the present- day rape, and afterward she was totally lost.

We have all gone through *sustos* during our lifetimes. Many of us have experienced many soul losses that have caused alterations, blocks, or holes within our energy body. When we do not express our anger, shock, abuse, and fright, it stays inside. When our spirit, the aura that surrounds us, is strong, our sacred soul—our essence, the root and core of who we really are—will not be deeply affected by the trials and tribulations of everyday life. One way of thinking of a healthy spirit is to compare it to the skin of a fruit. If the skin of the fruit is intact, it protects the fruit from bacteria and damage. If the skin is weakened or punctured, soon brown spots of decay begin to appear and spread throughout the fruit.

Espanto. Traditionally this disease describes the *susto* (fright) caused by seeing a ghost. According to Dr. Eliseo Torres in his book *The Folk Healer*, *espanto* can also occur when a person is asleep and is startled awake. Since at this time the spirit may have left the body to wander during dreams, it may not be close enough to return suddenly to the body. The causes of *espanto* include being awakened suddenly by something frightening such as a burglar, a disaster such as a fire or flood, by a fall from bed, or by a nightmare. Dr. Torres states that *espanto* can be more serious than *susto* because in *susto* the spirit may temporarily leave the body, but it does not go far. It can be persuaded to return to the body through a soul retrieval. In my culture, we use this term when we are surprised by someone. *Me espantaste!* "You frightened me!"

There is a belief that if one does not honor a deceased family member during Día de los Muertos (the Day of the Dead), his ghost will come back and haunt you. Día de los Muertos is a very important tradition. Every November 2 the dead are honored, as families make an altar for them decorated with flowers (usually marigolds), pictures of dead relatives, and their favorite foods, drinks, cigarettes, and candles. People believe that the smell of favorite foods and drinks will guide the spirit of a dead person back into this world to visit with his relatives and remind them that life and death are a natural part of the cycle of life. *Ofrendas*, altars and their offerings, are often also created at the cemetery. Día de los Muertos is an official holiday in Mexico and other Latin

American countries. I have seen cemeteries in Mexico full of families cooking food and making flower crosses over the headstone, as their children play among the dead. Mariachis sing songs, reminding listeners that our life here is brief.

I rarely treat *espanto*. Once in a while an individual will come to me complaining of sensing or seeing ghosts in her home, and wondering if her house is haunted. On such occasions, I will do a house blessing to change the vibration of the home. When a person is divorced or breaks up with the partner she has been living with, I also do a house blessing because a metaphorical death has occurred: the death of the relationship. The spirit of the spouse will stay in the house to "haunt" the person who has stayed behind.

Before I do a house blessing, I instruct my client to clean the house thoroughly, to pack up memories that are too painful, to rearrange the furniture, and to cover up the empty walls. In other words, I ask her to reclaim her house, heart, soul, and spirit. I also recommend that the person go through *luto*, one year of healing and grieving, before she gets involved with someone else.

Perhaps the true meaning of *espanto* is that it teaches us to take care of unfinished business. Perhaps ghosts visit us to request that we assist them in finishing whatever they must so that they can truly rest in peace. When I am treating my clients, I often dream of their departed loved ones. Most often, the dream takes the form of the deceased requesting that I give him or his family a *limpia*, a spiritual cleansing, because the deceased needs a "final closure" here on earth. We should not be afraid of ghosts. They have an important message for the living.

If we do not want ghosts to visit us, we should pay the dead their proper respect. When we pray "May he rest in peace," this prayer is also for the living. We need to take care of un- finished business because it will come back to haunt us if we don't.

Types of Curanderos and Their Specialties

Talking about types of curanderos or treatment specialties is not as easy as one might think. Even though scholarly articles and modern books on curanderismo divide curanderos into neat categories, in practice, curanderismo does not really work that way. Nevertheless, as a place to begin, I will talk about some of the standard definitions of the "types" of cu- randeros. I would like the reader to keep in mind, though, that curanderos often employ more than one of these cate- gories in their practice, and often use the tools of a particular category in unorthodox or individualized ways, depending on their personal style, training, and experience.

Hierbero — an herbalist. Not all curanderos are herbalists, but the majority of curanderos will use herbs in one way or an- other, whether as remedies for particular illnesses or in cleansing rituals such as *limpias* and sweat lodges. There are over eleven thousand catalogued healing herbs in the world today. Most curanderos feel that it is best to use whatever herbs are available in their local area, as herbs are most ef- fective when picked fresh. When I was sick with dysentery in Chalma, a town two hours south of Mexico City, my teacher Maestro Andres Segura did not pull an herb out of his medi- cine bag to cure me, but picked a plant locally.

Each culture has its own customs about the use of herbs, but most believe that the healer must have some sort of spiritual connection with the plants he or she uses. At the last Congress of Traditional Medicine in Guatemala, Aurelio Diaz, a medicine man of the Lakotas, said this about having a good relationship with healing herbs: "From your humility, *one plant* can help you cure people. The first medicine that was given to me cures everything. It is peyote. As I have traveled, I now have seven medicines." Many cultures believe that you can only use the herbs that have come to you in a dream or a vision, forming an alliance with you. Martín Prechtel, a shaman of the Tzutujil Maya Indians of Guatemala, knows something about the healing properties of over 600 herbs, but only uses the sixty or so that he has dreamed about. While I am not an herbalist, I personally grow the herbs that I use in my *limpias* and rituals: *ruda* (rue), *romero* (rosemary), and sage. In Mexico, besides *ruda* and *romero*, *pirul* (pepper tree) and *albacar* (sweet basil) are very popular. I could use other plants in my *limpias*, but I use *ruda* and *romero* because these plants grow where I live. I sweep bundles of herbs, and sometimes flowers, over a client's body to help remove sadness and energies that do not belong to him. To receive a *limpia* with a bunch of herbs or fresh flowers is pure pleasure.

Herbs are also used in sweat lodges as offerings to the spirits and to help with the healing and purification of the participants. In sweat lodges in the southwestern United States, people traditionally use sage, tobacco, lavender, cedar, and juniper. In Mexico, *romero*, *ruda*, and an aromatic plant with little white flowers called Santa Maria are used inside the sweat lodge. *Limpias* are commonly given to people within the lodge with the herb *pirul,* which is used because it has cosmic energy and harmonizes the body.

An herbalist does not pick herbs indiscriminately, but sees all plants as sacred, and will always make some kind of offering to the spirit of the plant he is harvesting—corn meal, tobacco, or a prayer. Healers make this offering because they know that there is always an exchange of energy between plants and the people who use them because plants are as alive as we are. They have much to teach us. As Aurielo Diaz reminded us at the congress, "To speak of the knowledge of our ancestors is to listen to the voice of the plants, the eagles, the wind, the dreams, and vision."

Sobadora—All curanderos have specific tools that they prefer, even though they may use many, depending upon what works best for them. The *sobadora* uses massage as her tool. Why do we need touch? Because all human beings require intimate contact. It has become popular for nursing schools today to offer courses in healing touch so that their graduates can know how to relax and soothe their patients when they are in pain, or when they just need reassurance. Curanderos use massage not only to relax the body and the muscles, but to touch the soul, to draw forth and begin to heal emotional and physical pain. They use it to help treat diseases such as *empacho* and *susto.* In my practice, I have found that we all have a universal need to be touched. When a client is frightened and anxious, I often have her lie down on my massage table. I use massage as a tool to help relieve her anxiety before I go any further with her. When working with the elderly, I always use massage, because the elderly in Western culture are almost always starved for touch.

We can see something of the dynamics behind massage—healing touch given by hands that love—in this story told to me by my Aztec teacher, Ehekateotl, who first learned massage from his mother. When Ehe was five years old, he liked to run out barefoot into the rain and get wet. This led to a chronic throat condition that eventually developed into rheumatic fever, which resulted in a physical weakness in his body from the waist down. His mother was able to heal him using a massage technique called *apapaxtli tlawayotl maihpahtli* that had been taught to her by Ehe's father.

"The blessed hands of my mother massaged my body from head to feet, touching the joints and tendons, muscles and bones, and she moved my entire body, causing me great pain. When I cried because my body was in great pain, she continued, giving me this treatment three times a day for three months until I could walk again. Western medical doctors told my parents that I would never walk, and now the most powerful part of my physical body is my legs, thanks to the care of my mother and the science of my father.

"I was massaged so often that I learned the therapy. But, in reality, it is not my hands that are working, but the extension of my mother's hands and the knowledge of my father. The technique is called, in Nahuatl, *apapaxtli*—in Spanish, *apapachar*—which commonly means 'expression of love,' but really means 'to soften.' *Tlawayotl* means 'what is generated from the heart of the people,' and *maihpahtli* signifies 'the hands that heal.' So the complete idea is 'to soften what the heart of the people generate with hands that heal.'"

For me, massage is a healing and diagnostic tool, as well as a way of helping my clients open up and tell me their stories more fully. On one occasion, I was visited by a man who told me that he was suffering from the ill effects of the *envídia* of his relatives who were living in Mexico. I was convinced that this was by no means the whole story, but I was having difficulty eliciting more information from this man, who, though very poor and very ill with a bronchial infection, was too proud to admit to his physical and emotional weakness. I decided to see if I could get further information on his problems by first helping him to relax his physical and emotional defenses through massage. Since he had just come from work and was still dressed in his work clothes, he apologized about not being as clean as he thought he should be, but I reassured him. I took off his work shoes and began to massage his feet, reaching, in this way, into all parts of his body, relaxing him and comforting a body that was starved for touch since his wife had left him recently. As I worked, he began to open up more and more, telling me parts of his story, until I was finally able to discover what was really troubling him.

Massage is not just the skillful physical manipulations of muscles to relieve pain and stress, but, in the hands of a curandero who understands the emotional, spiritual, and intuitive elements of massage, it can become a tool for further opening into the psyche. A curandero who gives the loving touch of massage feels no repulsion toward a body of any size, weight, or age—all are equally sacred as temples of the spirit.

Traditionally curanderos passed down this knowledge lovingly from parent to child. This passing down of knowledge through the family and apprentices is something that has been broken in modern times as indigenous peoples have been forced to assimilate into Western culture, but it is my hope that we will be able to begin to reclaim this way of teaching so that the knowledge of a lifetime of healing may not be lost. That is why I have taken on the training of apprentices at this time in my life. I once wrote about what receiving this kind of knowledge meant to me: "You sent me your seed through generations of ancestral grandmothers, and that seed is imbedded in the womb of my forever soul."

Partera — a curandera whose role is to be a midwife and provide pre- and postnatal care for a community. Traditionally, *parteras* were women who spent productive lives aiding in the birth of thousands of babies. One *partera* who was recently profiled on a New Mexican television station told viewers about her long and productive career. Now retired at the age of eighty-nine, she began studying *partera* at the age of thirteen, and has delivered twenty thousand babies, including twenty-five sets of twins and two sets of triplets, over the course of her career.

Parteras perform many useful and nurturing services for women, and there are many things that modern midwives, nurses, and doctors can learn from these traditional practices. I have visited many modern birthing centers that are remarkable, but I would like to encourage contemporary health care professionals to look at how *parteras* once nurtured the soul and emotions of the expectant mother. If I could encourage medical professionals to ask themselves one question, it would be: "What can I do in my practice to honor the spiritual beliefs of the mother?" In the old days, *parteras* were spokespersons for women and their needs. They were ritualists who prayed and lit candles on their altars for the safety of the mother and child, and baptized the baby as soon as it was born in case the infant died. If a child were born dead and deformed, they would not show the child to the mother, because they did not want her to become fearful of having another child. They would give her therapeutic reasons for the deformity so that the mother would not blame herself for her child's death. They might say, for example, "This child died because of the solar eclipse. It was not your fault that this happened."

These kinds of beliefs, for example, that a pregnant woman should not go outside during an eclipse of the sun or the moon, often sound strange to modern people. When I lecture to groups of women or health-care practitioners, often someone will ask me why *parteras* would counsel their clients not to go outside during an eclipse. I always admit that, while I don't honestly know the answer, I am not quite ready just to dismiss this belief as a superstition because there are so many indigenous cultures around the world that hold to this belief. For all I know, there could very well be some kind of scientific basis for it that we just haven't discovered yet. Once, in a moment of humorous inspiration, I asked the group I was addressing, "How many women in the audience are pregnant?" Several women raised their hands. I then asked, "And how many of you would go outside if there were an eclipse?" Not a single woman raised her hand. For that group, at least, it was better to be safe than sorry!

To me, one of the most incredible things that *parteras* did was to give a child a deep sense of place and belonging throughout his childhood. In the old days, the midwives would take the umbilical cord outside and bury it under a tree so that the child would always know that he was connected to the earth, and would always have a special tree all his own. It would make no sense for a modern midwife to do such a thing, but I feel it is important that we discover other rituals that make sense to us that can help children feel as if they belong to the community, and mothers feel comfortable and spiritually and emotionally cared for. That is the legacy that the *partera* can offer to modern midwives, doctors, and nurses.

Consejera — a counselor. Although all curanderos use *pláticas* (heart-to-heart talks) in their work, *consejeras* are those who specialize in counseling clients on anything that they might want to talk about: shyness, relationship and marital problems, difficulties with children, health problems, fears that one has been hexed, job problems, envy, grief and loss, etc. Curanderos make great counselors for many reasons. In a world where many medical doctors seldom give a patient more then a few minutes to answer the question "How do you feel?" *consejeras* give their patients all the time in the world. *Consejeras* keep hours that make it easy for working people to seek out their services. They usually work out of their homes, and will sit you down, make you comfortable, and fix you a soothing cup of tea. They will never cut you off or look at the clock when you are trying to tell them something about yourself.

Although *consejeras* do many of the same things that psychotherapists do, it is not really accurate to label them as such. A modern psychotherapist is someone who has been trained in one or more particular schools, such as Jungian or Rogerian psychology, and most of the time adheres to the rules and framework of her training school when counseling patients. For example, a Rogerian therapist is trained not to dialogue with a patient, but rather to mirror every statement back to the client by saying something like, "What do *you* think about that?" Modern therapists are taught that it is seldom wise to get overly emotionally involved with their clients or to offer direct advice. Like medical doctors, their responses to their patients are sometimes shaped by a fear of malpractice suits.

Although I am not exclusively a *consejera, pláticas* and counseling are certainly among my most important healing modalities. The many years I spent working as a psychiatric nurse, following guidelines and protocols of treatment that often seemed inadequate and rigid, have given me a lasting appreciation for the creative and flexible approach of the *consejera*. In particular, I remember the years I spent as a clinical nurse specialist at UCLA at the Neuropsychiatric Institute working with emotionally disturbed children between the ages of seven and eleven. Although this was the best hospital I had ever worked at, and my position there was prestigious, I felt a great deal of frustration with the treatment guidelines we had to follow. For example, we were never permitted to reinforce negative behavior, no matter what the children did or said to us. This led to some very emotionally trying situations for all of the counselors and nurses. Some of the children we were treating were psychotic. Others had come from abusive homes and were used to acting out verbally and physically. On one occasion, when one of the children spit on me, calling me a "dirty Mexican," I just had to sit and take it because getting angry or correcting a child for acting out was considered "reinforcing negative behavior." Finding positive behaviors that I could reinforce were few and far between, and I often found myself thinking, "But I don't get this. It isn't working." I could not see how this rule was really benefiting the children because, in the real world, it is unrealistic to expect that negative behavior does not have consequences. What I really saw was a staff that was "stuffing" its feelings, and children learning unrealistic ways to behave.

Finally one day I was counseling a young boy who kept giving me the finger and saying, "Fuck you," every time I asked him if he was ready to go to school. After telling him, "Okay, I'll be back in three minutes. Please be ready," I was greeted by an especially violent "Fuck you" and a hand gesture shoved in my face as the boy lunged forward. Looking down at the boy's feet, and at a loss as to what I could possibly say that sounded the least bit positive, I said, "Look, you've taken your first step forward." Later on, in the counselor's lounge, I told my colleagues, "All right, I get it. I found something positive to say. But what good did that do?"

Unlike traditional therapists, the *consejera* does not have to follow a protocol about what she can and can't say or do. She will follow her heart, her intuition, and whatever divine guidance she adheres to. For this reason, *consejeras* are often able to be more expansive and interactive with their clients than Western mental-health workers. The technique employed by the consejera is called *desahogar*, which means that the client speaks until *everything* has been released from the body, soul, and heart. During this process, the heart of the *consejera* will be equally engaged. As Aurelio, the Lakota medicine man who spoke at the Twelfth Congress of Traditional Medicine, said, *"Corazón cura corazón."* Heart cures heart.

If a patient cries during a session with a modern therapist, she usually does it sitting alone in her chair. A *consejera* will not be afraid to cradle you while you grieve, or let you cry on her shoulder. She is not afraid of the healing power of touch. She might sing you a lullaby, or chant for you while she gently drums, or take you to her altar and pray with you. One thing is sure, she will help you feel better.

Nor is the *consejera* afraid of allowing people the freedom of other forms of emotional expression. How many people would feel comfortable screaming in their therapist's office? The receptionist might hear, or the next patient waiting in the adjacent room, or the person in the office next door. When I had my garage remodeled into a treatment room, one of the things I made sure of was that there was enough soundproofing to offer my clients the privacy to release their most painful emotions. Many people live with an agony of grief or pain that they have been holding inside for years.

People also tell *consejeras* things that they might be afraid to tell a traditional therapist, things that they consider too weird, frightening, or bizarre. If a client tells a *consejera* that he is hearing voices, or that he fears that someone is psychically attacking him with *envidia* or has put a curse on him, the *consejera* will not judge. A *consejera* does not put you into a straitjacket and cart you off to an institution if you tell her your most terrible thoughts. She will not send you to a psychiatrist who will fill you up with psychiatric drugs that are supposed to return you to "normal."

Another difference between modern therapists and *consejeras* is the type of history that each takes. A therapist, nurse, or psychiatrist may spend two or three sessions taking a patient's history, but the questions that are usually asked during such an assessment are limited by the parameters of traditional medicine. A *consejera* brings more creativity to the questions she asks. She is not barred from asking patients about their spiritual belief system, or the condition of their soul, nor does she ever leave out the day-to-day social aspects of what might be troubling a person. A *consejera* might ask, "Are you having money problems? How are your kids doing in school? Have you been getting along all right with your in-laws?" As the treatment progresses, she might ask, "What kind of values or belief systems are you holding on to? Have any of these beliefs ceased to serve you? If so, would you like to let go of any of them?"

I often make use of this kind of creative questioning, intuition, and sensitivity when I am working with a new client. Once a woman came to see me who was complaining of health problems. She had been to a lot of doctors, but none of them had been able to help her. I have found that many of the women who come to me have unresolved issues about abortions, so I always make it part of my initial interview to ask a woman if she has ever had an abortion. Sensing that this woman was in deep grief over something, I asked her this question and she immediately began to cry. She revealed that she had gone to a psychic several months ago who had told her that the child she was pregnant with would be born deformed and urged her to abort it. Panicked, the woman had complied. Since then, she had been filled with a deep horror and grief at what she had done.

I made an appointment for her to come back and have a *limpia*. When she returned, she told me that this was the exact day that her child would have been born. Using the creativity of the *consejera*, I simply made this date part of our ceremony. I sensed that the woman was grieving because she could not forgive herself for what she had done, so I put my hand on her womb and told her that she had to go through the birthing process in order to be able to let go of the child finally. At times like these, I can feel divine guidance moving through me, guiding my actions. I had the woman lie down on my massage table, put her legs in the birthing position, and began massaging her stomach, leading her through the entire process of having the child. I asked her to remember the moment of conception, to feel the child grow month by month in her body, and then, finally, to push the child out of her birth canal into the world. I asked her to give the child a name and a gender, and then to let it go. As the woman wept and said good-bye to the doll I had asked her to bring to represent the child, she was finally able to let go of the heavy burden she had been carrying around inside of her and begin a grieving process that was healing and liberating.

When I worked as a traditional therapist or as a psychiatric nurse, I used to feel bored taking a patient's history. As a curandera, I find myself looking forward with excitement to each new patient's story. As I listen to my patients open their hearts, I ask myself the question, "Where is this story going to go and how is divine energy going to manifest as the two of us cocreate this patient's healing together?" What used to be dull, uniform, and frustrating has become an exciting journey of mystery, creativity, and vibrant healing.

Espiritualista—a trance medium. Curanderos who are *espiritualistas* are not very common anymore in the United States, although many curanderos feel, at one time or another, as if they are channeling certain energies or receiving information from the spiritual realm. According to what Trotter and Chavira write in their book *Curanderismo: Mexican American Folk Healing,* the work of the *espiritualista*

> ... revolves around a belief in spirit beings who inhabit another plane of existence, but who are interested in making periodic contacts with the world. The curandero learns to become a link, a direct line of communication between this and that other world. The heart of the spiritual movement in Mexican American communities lies in the activities of spiritual centers that are staffed by trance mediums. Mediumship is the ability to act as a communicating link with the spiritual world.

In Mexico, there is a large group of *espiritualistas* called *Fidencistas* who channel one of the most famous curanderos of all time, Niño Fidencio, a healer who is considered by many to be a folk saint. According to Dr. Torres in his book, *Folk Healers,* Fidencio was born in Guanajuato, Mexico, in 1898. He began performing cures when he was eight years old and continued until his death at the age of forty. A childlike, happy man who earned the nickname of El Niño (The Child), he often prescribed laughter, food, and merriment to the many people who came to consult with him. When anyone gave him gifts, El Niño would use the occasion to share, thus lightening the otherwise gloomy existence of many of the pilgrims who came to see him. He often hired musicians and encouraged everyone, even arthritics and cripples, to dance. He was so famous for his cures that even today, sixty years after his death, thirty thousand people from all over the United States and Mexico make the pilgrimage to his birthplace at Espinoza, Mexico, twice a year to pay homage to him. The *Fidencistas*, his followers who channel his healing energy, dress in white shirts and red kerchiefs and are said to assume his very spirit. They are believed actually to become El Niño while they are in a trance state.

When I go into a trance while working with a client, I do not channel a particular entity, but I often feel as if knowledge from God is coming through me. This divine energy tells me what to say and do to create an opening for a healing to occur. I always begin my rituals by calling that divine energy in, inviting it to be present with myself and my patients.

While I was in Durango, Mexico, recently I visited an *espiritualista* named Hermano José, who channels a very old Indian spirit. He took my hand and went immediately into trance, telling me many things about myself. He said, "There are many people who are envious of you, and there are also people who come to you, not for healing, but to observe you." A traditional curandero, he began by rubbing an egg over my body, and then chanted some traditional prayers. He took me to an adjoining room with a cement floor, poured alcohol on the floor, and started a big fire. Taking two huge bunches of *ruda* and *romero*, he passed them through the fire clockwise and then passed them over me, giving me a *limpia*, telling me to release all of my negativity to the fire. Then he prescribed special baths and prepared two candles on which he scratched my name in the wax. Lastly he gave me an amulet for protection. Like many traditional curanderos, Hermano José sees many people, sometimes up to sixty per day.

Huesero — similar to a chiropractor. Someone who does spinal adjustments and sets dislocated joints. In the United States, with the advent of modern medicine, this type of curandero has almost disappeared.

The Curandero Total—A *curandero total* is a healer who employs all four of the levels of medicine described by my Aztec teacher, Ehekateotl: education, bodywork, medicine, and sacred tools. This is true holistic medicine because all four of these techniques involve the soul and spirit of the healer and his patient. To Ehe, the curandera's first and most important tool is her knowledge. Educating her patients on taking responsibility for their health is the most important message she can convey. Healthy habits and customs include learning how to breathe, rest, hydrate, and eat properly. *Pláticas* with the curandera comprise part of this education.

The second level of treatment is bodywork. This might involve the "laying on of hands," *sobadas*, *apapaxtli* (the Aztec technique of massage), Rolfing, or simply touching with compassion. The body is a door to the soul and spirit. The body does not lie.

The third level is "the medicine," which includes plants, minerals, animals, and the gases that they produce, and the proper handling of these medicines.

The last level is what Ehe calls the "tools of the trade." These tools can be the feathers, crystals, and the branches of flowers or plants, such as *romero*, that are swept over a patient's body to remove unwanted energies during a *limpia*. They can include human-made instruments such as stethoscopes, X-rays, or sonograms, and sound makers such as drums and musical instruments.

Ehekateotl is a *curandero total*. He and all my compadres and comadres from his teaching center, the Centro de Desarrollo Cultural Tetzkatlipoka Kallulli (Cultural Development Center of the Smoky Mirror), are my friends, teachers, and relatives. My own apprenticeship currently involves learning more about herbology and massage. Maybe someday I will be a *curanðera total.* I am still learning.

In 1997 when Ehekateotl was visiting me in New Mexico, he advised me to wrap up my *ðahumaðor* (incense burner) and return it to my previous teacher, Andres Segura. I had disobeyed Segura and Ehe felt that I should return this tool to him with an apology. I knew he was right. Maestro Segura had asked me not to take my *ðahumaðor* outside my healing room, and I had disobeyed out of ignorance and arrogance.

Knowing that I would have to give back this important tool, I went through a deep grieving for several days. During this time, Ehe was kind to me and helped open me up to a deeper understanding of the medicine that he was teaching me. He asked me, "If you cannot use your *ðahumaðor* and burn your copal, what other tools do you have?"

"I have my egg, my eagle feather, and my *romero,*" I replied sadly. I felt so lost without my *ðahumaðor.*

"If you did not have your eagle feather, egg, and romero?"

"I would have my hands," I said.

"If you did not have your hands?" he prodded.

I went deeper. "I would have my heart," I whispered.

"Now you realize that the tools we get so attached to are not as important as our heart," he said.

I understood his teaching and I felt a sense of peace. I realized that, over the past twenty years that I have been practicing this medicine, my compassion, my soul, and a sincere desire to be of service have been all that I have really needed.

A few days later, Ehe and Tzen invited me into my healing

room. There they asked me to join them in a ceremony in which they handed me my new *sahumador.* What a profound and loving way to learn the true meaning of being a curandera!

There are many creative ways to view illness and health, just as there are many creative ways to heal or manage disease. Too often in Western medicine, medical treatments are shrouded in scientific jargon and mystery. How can we take responsibility for our health if our healers hide behind medical language, pedestals, or barriers that keep us from understanding our illness? My hope is that healers and health practitioners begin to accept their responsibility to educate people, helping them to discover their own inner healing and medicine. All human beings have medicine inside of us—we have the ability to cure ourselves—and every person's illness is unique. It is my hope that the healers of the future will help people to find the medicine that is right for them, and not what the healer thinks is right for them.

Chapter Two

Doctora Corazón
The Training of a Curandera

When I was a little girl growing up in El Paso, Texas, my mother and I loved to listen to a daily radio program from Mexico called *Doctora Corazón,* "Doctor of the Heart." This was a call-in show that invited people to share their problems with the *doctora.* As people told her about their difficulties with their children, romantic conflicts, loneliness, marriage problems, and broken hearts, the *doctora* would give them advice. Listening to all these sorrows, my little heart used to open up with compassion. These difficulties seemed insurmountable, and I would listen in amazement as the *doctora* always came up with what seemed like incredible solutions.

When people talk about curanderismo, they often say that healers must study, but they must also be born with the *don*, the "healing gift." Just as young musicians will pound on the piano and beat on pots and pans, and young future veterinarians will rescue sick animals and doctor all the creatures in the neighborhood, gifted healers long from a very young age to alleviate the pain and suffering they see around them. As I became more and more fascinated with the therapeutic magic of Doctora Corazón, I began to practice giving advice to the neighborhood kids, much like Lucy in the Peanuts cartoon with her sign, The Psychiatrist Is In. In my neighborhood, the *consejera* was always in.

If any of the local kids needed help, I would be there, ready to offer solutions, often whether they wanted my advice or not, sometimes with hilarious results. When I was fourteen, I had a friend named Sammy who was two or three years older and had terrible acne. He always confided in me about how sad he felt that no girl wanted to date him because of his face. Feeling a great deal of sympathy for Sammy, I told him that I had once heard that having sexual relations was a good cure for acne. A month later, Sammy came back to me, furious. He had followed my advice and gone over the border to Juárez, Mexico, where he had slept with a prostitute and picked up a bad case of syphilis that required a large and painful shot of penicillin. About a week later, however, his acne miraculously cleared up. I didn't realize it at the time, but I had inadvertently pointed him in the right direction since antibiotics are one of the few cures that work with acute acne. In spite of occasional missteps such as this, the neighborhood kids continued to trust me and to come to me for advice.

I also developed an early love for the mysteries of ceremony and ritual. As the "neighborhood priest," I would plan elaborate weddings on Saturday afternoons, choosing who would be the bride; who would play the roles of groom, flower girl, bridesmaids, and ushers; and who would be the choir and sing the bridal march while the wedding party marched down the aisle. Everything had to be perfect, and I would go through my mom's clothes and steal or beg whatever I could to dress for the part. Because there were no flowers in my apartment complex, I also learned which *señoras* in the neighborhood grew the best blossoms, and gave the other kids directions about where to steal them.

While I was acting as mother, counselor, and priest to the other children in the neighborhood, I did not always feel that I was receiving enough of the kind of love I needed at home. The second to the eldest in a family of six girls and one boy, and a very sensitive and needy child, I seldom got as much attention as I craved from my parents. My mother, a proud, beautiful, and high-strung woman who had been born into an upper-class family in Mexico, hated the poverty and the abuse that she received from her husband, my father, when he was on one of his alcoholic binges. She did not like for my five sisters and me to play with the neighborhood kids because they were "peasants." We Martinez girls would get rocks thrown at us by some of these kids who felt we were snobs.

My mother was engaged in a daily struggle to keep up appearances while coping with the grim realities of poverty. She somehow found the money to send all six of her daughters to private schools and to sew us beautiful wardrobes that lived up to her expectations of how her children should be dressed. But as the years passed, this constant effort to make one plus one add up to ten took its toll on her spirit.

My father, a tall, handsome, and deeply intelligent individual, also wrestled with his own private demons. A man who had never had the money or opportunity to follow his dream of being an engineer, he had worked for over thirty years as a mechanic at the local army base, humbly calling white men "sir" all day long. My father coped with his lost dreams by periodically going on alcoholic binges. Because of my innate sensitivity, I was able to predict accurately which paydays my father would come home drunk. Every Friday, my sisters would anxiously ask me what condition I thought our papa would be in when he came through the door, and I would give them an answer based upon the condition of my stomach. If Papa had been drinking, my stomach ached, and we were all in for a rough evening.

Because of my sensitivity to the upheavals and unhappiness that sometimes went on in my home, I became a thin and sickly child whose nickname was Huecitos, "Little Bones." Worried about my poor health and constant stomachaches, my mother was always using her store of *remedios* to try to help her daughter gain weight and feel better. In many ways, my mother was the perfect person to raise a daughter who would become a curandera. Even though she was sometimes exasperated with a child who was so sickly and demanded so much attention, I learned a lot about curing from receiving my mother's ministrations, and my mother and I formed a bond through the many teas that she so conscientiously gave me to drink. I was dosed with *yerba buena* (peppermint leaves) for my stomach, and *manzanilla* (chamomile) to help me sleep. I did not like to be touched by my mother because she was often physically abusive, which made me feel that I could not trust her touch, but she would show me how to massage my own stomach when I had *empacho*. My mother also knew how to treat simple *susto* in her children by giving us sugar water when one of us saw something upsetting. Once when I saw a dog run over by a car and ran inside the house crying, my mother mixed a teaspoon of sugar in a glass of water and made me drink it. Modern health-care professionals know that one of the most useful treatments for mild shock is dextrose, a form of sugar.

My mother often called in one of the local curanderas when something happened to one of her children that she couldn't cure. When my older sister Irma, who was a very pretty child, suffered from frequent bouts of *mal ojo* due to the constant attention she was receiving from strangers, my mother would ask a curandera to do a ceremony for her. I always had terrible attacks of envy when this happened and I used to complain to my mother about all of the attention that my sister was getting. "Aren't I pretty enough to get *mal ojo?*" I would ask.

"Don't be envious!" my mother would say in exasperation to this daughter who was always trying to get her attention. Not surprisingly, this made me, who secretly despaired that I was not as pretty, not as good, and not as talented as my adorable and much-doted-upon sister, feel terrible—especially because no one made any effort to arrange a ceremony to cure me of my envy.

I grew up in the barrio of El Paso, Texas, where my family lived in a presidio, a block-long building that looked something like a military garrison and housed between fifteen and twenty families. Each apartment had three rooms, a living room, bedroom, and kitchen, and a small porch that led to the backyard and communal outhouse. The backyard was a wide strip of dirt that contained neither trees, grass, nor flowers.

A very sensual little girl, I loved kicking sand with my bare feet and jumping into puddles, and got a lot of pleasure out of just about anything that got me wet and muddy. When it rained, I would run down the streets and splash in all the mud puddles, feeling joyously carefree and getting unbelievably filthy in the process. Dirt didn't bother me because I was in love with the earth. Sometimes I would mix earth and water to make mud, rubbing it all over myself, reveling in the fresh smell. When it got dark and my mother forced me to come inside the house, all I wanted to do was to crawl into bed, content with the cozy sleepy feeling that comes from playing in the dirt all evening. Unfortunately my mother would force me to get into the bathtub and wash my feet before I went to bed. She often spanked me for getting the sheets full of dirt, and my sisters, who shared the bed with me, did not appreciate it either. Nor was that the end of my indignities. *"Mójate la mollera,"* my mother would yell from the kitchen, "Wet the top of your head." I would do what she asked, but I would feel as if this were an insult to my young spirit, and I would go to bed, night after night, furious with her.

The desert around my home grew many aromatic plants, such as the creosote bush that releases sharp piney incense after it rains. At such times, when my senses were filled to the brim with the spiritual fragrances of the desert, my young soul would become intoxicated and I would have to be dragged struggling into the house at the end of the day. This also exasperated my mother, who perhaps did not recognize her own expansive, romantic, and dramatic soul mirrored in her daughter.

True to the Nahuatl name Xochitl, meaning "flower," that I would be gifted with later in life, I loved flowers and, since I always knew the location of the most beautiful ones in the neighborhood, my sisters made me the official flower thief for Mother's Day. I spent many hours lying on my back on the warm earth, looking up at the expansive daytime and night-time skies of El Paso, which boasted magnificent sunrises and sunsets over the mountains that surrounded the town. It was as if, lacking sufficient love and attention from human parents, I made all of nature my mother.

A curandera, especially one who does soul retrievals, knows the importance of names. If the true name of a person is not known, it will be difficult or impossible to call back the part of the soul that is absent. The soul is literally anchored to our name. Born Ada Elena Martinez (Ada was also my mother's name), I "lost" my first name when I went to kinder-garten at the Guardian Angel School. There the nuns Angli-cized the pronunciation of my first name, Ada, and the kids began to call me Aida. It was also a strange feeling not to be called by the name Elena (or Elenita) that I was known by at home.

At age eleven, I lost my second name. I became very ill one night and woke up the next morning in the county hospital. Too sick with hepatitis to be aware of my surroundings, I was terrified by the sounds and smells of the hospital, and the pokings and intrusions into my body. It was the first time I had ever been away from home, and the nurses and doctors on the seventh floor, who were loving and cheerful, became my new family. I believe that my desire to become a nurse was born, in part, from the compassion and validation they gave to me. They changed my name to Helen because it was easier for them to pronounce, and encouraged me to drink large quantities of milk to strengthen my liver.

Because I was lactose intolerant, the milk made me even sicker. One evening when my mother was visiting, I became so ill that I began throwing up violently, the milk spraying out of me like a projectile. I was terrified that my mother would be angry with me, but she wasn't. She was so tender and attentive that I began to believe that I was going to die, and that this was the only reason my mother was being so patient with me as I made this horrible mess all over her, the bed, and the floor. At that point, in my child's mind, I began to reason that if dying was the price I had to pay for my mother's attention, it was no longer safe to have a mother. From that time on, I made a decision that I had to be totally self-sufficient if I wanted to survive. I told my family to call me Helen from then on, a name I would carry for twenty-seven years until I reclaimed my identity.

In my desire to escape from a home life that was becoming increasingly turbulent, I married very early, at age sixteen. My first child, Jamie, was born when I was seventeen, and I spent the next decade and a half trying to give my children everything I felt that I hadn't received myself. As my family absorbed more and more of my energies, my fascination with healing had to be pretty much put on hold for years. Even if my life hadn't been so busy, it is unlikely that it would ever have occurred to me to study curanderismo. During the 1940s through the 1970s, Chicanos were feeling a tremen-

dous pressure to assimilate into mainstream American culture, and things such as curanderismo were considered passé
and old-fashioned. I was swept along by those currents.

My talent for healing did receive some encouragement in
my early twenties. When I began working as a receptionist
for three gynecologists, my natural curiosity and hunger to
learn led me to ask the doctors and Rose Tarin, the RN who
worked in the office, a lot of questions about the practice of
medicine. As I learned to read charts and became proficient
in understanding medical procedures, Rose told me that I
had a natural talent for healing and would make a great
nurse. Without realizing it, she was handing me, a young
woman who hadn't even finished high school, one of the most
important gifts I would ever receive: a belief in myself and the
importance of what I loved. I never forgot her words. Six
years later, I earned my GED in night school, and began four
years of full-time study at the University of Texas at El Paso
where I earned my bachelor's in nursing.

Tragically, three weeks before my graduation, my mother
committed suicide by taking an overdose of antidepressants.
This was devastating for me, because I had wanted more than
anything in the world for her to see me graduate. She had
been so proud of my decision to get my GED and go to college, and had bragged to all her friends that her daughter was
studying to be a doctor. When I had corrected her, saying,
"Mom, I'm not in medical school, I'm studying nursing," she
had replied, "So what's the difference?" My graduation ceremony was supposed to be the event that would vindicate me,
that would prove, for all time, that the wild and difficult child
I had once been had grown into a woman who really was

"good enough." As it turned out, it was one of the most miserable nights of my life. I received my degree in 1976 and earned my master's in 1981.

Ironically, it was my very desire to assimilate by earning a professional degree that started me on my path to rediscovering the medicine of my heritage. During my first year of nursing school, in 1972, one of my professors asked me to do a report on curanderismo. At the time, there was a big movement to go back to holistic nursing and cultural health-care values. Because I was one of the few Chicanas in the program, the teacher just assumed that I could get up and rattle off all the folk diseases and cures and enlighten everyone in the class about curanderismo.

For me, this request brought up a lot of self-doubt and worry. I had been working so hard to assimilate, and was the first person in my family to receive a college degree. Full of big plans and big dreams for my future, I wanted to lose my accent and be like every other professional in mainstream American culture. When the professor asked me to talk about curanderismo, I felt ashamed, insulted, and bewildered. What was it that she saw about me? I wondered. Did she see my ignorance, the superstitions of my culture? Over the years, I had come to associate curanderismo with everything that was primitive and backward.

Since there was no way out of this embarrassing situation, I went to the library with the intent of reading a couple of articles and bullshitting the class. Instead, something profound happened. In the quiet, scientific atmosphere of the school of nursing library, I found tangible evidence of my mother's love and her attempts to nurture her wayward daughter:

Mal aire (bad air) is a disease that manifests with cold symptoms, ear aches, or facial paralysis. It can be prevented by not staying outside after dusk, covering a baby from the night air, and, if the body gets wet, achieving balance by wetting the top of the head. *Mal aire* comes from too much exposure to the evening air.

Reading this brief, lackluster description of *mal aire* in a monograph, I was suddenly, magically transported back into my childhood. I heard my mother calling to me, *"Mójate la mollera."* "Wet the top of your head." Between the lines of that dry, academic description, I began to discover my own memories, the story of how much my mother had cared for my health. Suddenly I was struck by a memory of myself as a young girl playing in the dirt in the evening, rolling on the ground with the other children, and loving the smell of the earth. I heard my mother calling out to me at five-minute intervals, "It's almost time to come into the house," and then finally insisting that I come in because it was getting dark. When my mother told me to take a bath, I hadn't wanted to get clean, to take the delicious fragrance of the earth from my body. So I would try for a compromise, "Can't I just wash my feet?" and my mother would answer, "Okay, but wet the top of your head."

As I read the "scientific" explanation of how wetting the top of the head after wetting one's extremities made it possible for the body to keep its temperature homeostatically in balance, I realized with a pang how much my mother must have loved me. Even though the child Elenita had gone to bed angry, night after night, because her mother had insisted that she wash herself and put water on her head, the adult Elena finally understood that my mother had been watching over my health, protecting me from *mal aire*.

As I paged through other descriptions of the diseases treated by curanderismo, I was flooded with memories I hadn't touched on in years. As I read the short description of *susto*, I remembered my mother mixing up sugar water for me and my sisters when we witnessed something that made us upset. I recalled how the beautiful Irma had gotten *mal ojo* from all the people who admired her, and how little Elenita had suffered the pangs of *envidia*. I felt sad for that little girl that no one thought was pretty, and who had not received a special ceremony to cure the envy that made her heart ache. Here was my culture, sitting in black-and-white on the page of a monograph; and, because I had lived it, all of these things rose living and vibrant off the page. Something inside of me stirred and began to come awake.

I gave my report to the class that week, but I also decided that the curanderismo of my childhood had value and was worth further study. Since all nursing students had to do assessments on patients, and since there was a strong focus on holistic nursing at that time, I decided that it would be all right for me to conduct some of my own field research on curanderismo at the hospital. I continued to ask the usual questions about patients' physical, psychological, emotional, and socio-economic status; but I also began to incorporate questions about their cultural beliefs. For example, if someone broke his leg under really traumatic circumstances, I would ask him if he felt that he had suffered any *susto*.

When I began writing these kinds of questions and answers up in my reports, most of my instructors were happy to have this information, since it also enhanced their own cultural knowledge. One professor, however, told me in no uncertain terms to stop focusing so much on "all this cultural stuff." I was crushed. As happens so often, I heard only the negative feedback and started worrying about whether or not I was getting what my professors were teaching me in the courses. I still asked my patients about curanderismo, but I began to focus more strongly on the "official" questions and write up my reports in the standard way.

The professor who criticized the way I was writing my assessments could not stop the growing trend in the medical profession toward transcultural nursing. As my knowledge of curanderismo grew, I began to get calls from hospitals and other organizations to come and give brief lectures on the subject. These requests for lectures on curanderismo had begun even when I was still a nursing student. Once I had graduated and was working as a psychiatric nurse, they came even more often. When I had exhausted the literature that the libraries had to offer, I began to visit curanderos and curanderas in El Paso and over the border in Juárez, Mexico, to see what I could learn from them. At first I told myself that I was just doing more research, but I had already started down what I would later begin to call my path of healing, the journey to heal my own wounds. I started becoming aware of the tremendous amount of pain that I had to heal in my life. I needed to heal the pain of my mother's death, my father's alcoholism, my many childhood illnesses, a terrifying near-death experience I had at age fifteen when I had almost drowned, my feelings of not being pretty enough, and my envy of my beautiful sister. I also realized that some of the greatest scars that I carried came from the racism I had experienced, the many put-downs of my cultural beliefs, such as my teacher's warnings that I should not write any more about curanderismo in my assessments. There had been many doors closed in my face, both literally and figuratively, because I was a Chicana. Once when my husband and I were looking for apartments in San Angelo, Texas, a woman had slammed the door on us, saying, "We don't rent apartments to Mexicans!" This terrible experience had cut deeply; especially since I was only seventeen at the time, and my husband was doing his service to his country in the air force. What had begun as a search for information was fast becoming a journey to healing and self-transformation. I did not know it then, but the *desarrollo,* the training, of a curandera would force me, as a wounded healer, to search for my own wholeness.

It was not hard to find curanderos and curanderas to learn from. Even though some Chicanos in the United States were trying to assimilate and forget "all that stuff," curanderismo was vibrantly alive in Mexico. I went to Mexico to learn about curanderismo because the root was still there and the culture was still intact. In Juárez, I went to the *mercado,* the store where herbs, flowers, special healing soaps and candles, and statues of saints were sold. I learned from the healers I found working there by telling them my problems and listening to the questions they asked me, their knowledge, the stories that they would share. I soon began to realize that these were not ignorant, uneducated people, but individuals with a deep therapeutic understanding of human behavior, the energies of the body, the use of herbs, and the mysteries of human experience. In many cases, I was impressed with the profound subtleties of the counsel that I received. For example, one curandera suggested, after giving me a *limpia,* that I also

give my house a spiritual cleansing. By this time, I was working as a nurse on the psychiatric floor of a local hospital.
Without realizing it, I had been bringing home the energy of
the anguish and pain of the psychiatric patients. The curandera told me how to cleanse by house by burning charcoal in
a brazier, carrying it to the corners of each room, and saying
special prayers.

Unfortunately this was a bit too much for my family, who
had been patiently humoring me along as I studied this
"weird stuff." While I was doing the cleansing ceremony in
my home, holding the smoking charcoal brazier in one hand
and my sheet of prayers in the other, my son Jamie began to
roll on the floor laughing. "Mom, this time you've finally lost
it." Because of the teasing, head shaking, and bewildered reactions my friends and family expressed when I tried to talk
to them about the ceremonies and practices I was discovering, I decided that I needed to be more circumspect. In spite
of everything, however, I was unwilling to stop learning. The
things that the curanderos were telling me made perfect sense
to me. If people could benefit from clearing unwanted energies from their bodies to help keep them in good health, why
should it not make just as much sense to remove unwanted
energies from their homes to make the place where they lived
a safe and nurturing space?

As I continued my explorations, I also began to realize
that, as in all professions, there were some curanderos who
were only in it for the money they could make off desperate
and gullible people. As I began to discriminate more and
more, I realized that the curanderos that I felt drawn to the
most were the ones who included me in the ceremony that accompanied my treatment, whatever that might be. I began to

steer clear of those who predicted catastrophes, and even future events. While I believe that some individuals were genuinely able to see into the future, I am equally convinced that human beings benefit most by solving their own problems, and not being handed the answers in the form of precognitive advice.

One of my most powerful experiences at this time involved my first soul retrieval. On this occasion, I told a curandera about how I had almost drowned in Acapulco when I was fifteen. The healer explained to me that the emptiness and fear that I felt while remembering this experience was a symptom of severe *susto*. Leading me to her very beautiful altar, she told me that she was going to ask God to be present and to help her bring back that part of my soul that had stayed in the ocean during those moments when I was deep under the water, sure that I was going to die. She gave me a *limpia* with a bundle of herbs, and swept my body with a small hand broom made from soft grasses. Then she blew some of her breath into the top of my head, and put her mouth to my ear, softly calling my name. She did not call for "Helen," but "Elenita," the loving diminutive of my real name. "Elenita, Elenita, *regresa*," she said, which means "come back." After this experience, I was filled with peace and truly felt that something within me had healed. I knew that I needed and wanted more—and more. Soon the local curanderos were not enough and I began going into the interior of Mexico.

Even though I was happier following this path, my family was becoming very concerned about the many changes they saw happening in me. My father came from a generation that had internalized the judgment of the dominant white culture that curanderismo was backward and primitive. Now he saw his daughter, his hope, the first person in his family to get a college education and achieve the dream of success that he'd always had, going back to her indigenous roots, and this worried him. At one point, he asked me, *"Mijita, why do you want to become an Indian?"*

"Because I am," I answered him.

"But you have French blood and Spanish blood."

"I know, but I want to honor my roots."

My children were also puzzled at this turn my life had taken. From the time I had quit high school to get married until the time when my older children were in early adolescence, my whole life had been devoted to them. The life I had provided for them had been very stable and I had worked hard at being a very traditional Chicana wife and mother. I'd taken them faithfully to mass on Sundays, celebrated holidays and birthdays with *piñatas* and traditional meals for the whole family and all our friends, and chauffeured them to Brownies and Little League. Even while I was working on my GED and then going to night school to get my college degree, my children had always come first.

Then all of a sudden I began to travel to Mexico, dress in *huipiles* and huaraches, and do weird stuff like house cleansings. Everything changed further when I divorced their father in 1977. By this time my older children, Jamie and Sondie, were fifteen and thirteen, and the twins, Abel and Adrian, were six. The maid had to be let go, and the house and most of the material possessions had to be sold off to pay the bills when the estate was divided between my husband and me, and the kids were angry that they had lost their big house and the good life. El Paso is a pretty conservative place where success means material possessions and getting out of the barrios. They would say to me, "Mom, why are you so weird? Why can't you be like all the other mothers?" I knew that I had swallowed the myth of the perfect mother and wife, but I couldn't digest it. My soul was desperate to find itself and I felt I would wither and die if I returned to my old way of being. The older kids decided to stay with their father, and the twins, who had been going to ceremonies with me since they were young, stayed with me.

As I traveled deeper into Mexico, I not only found more curanderos to learn from, I began to discover my roots, my culture, and my soul. My mother had been a woman of Mayan and Spanish descent whose parents spoke their tribal language and had originally immigrated to the U.S. from Mérida in the region of the Yucatán. My father had been born in San Juan del Rio Durango, in northern Mexico, and his genetic mixture was Zapotec, Aztec, and European. Even though I am biologically a mestiza, I realized that I knew very little about the history of my people. This history had not been taught in my schools, nor had my parents shared it with me because they were too busy trying to assimilate and survive. I began to learn stories of the Conquest told, not through the eyes of the Europeans, but through the eyes of my people. One very important story that I learned was the tale of Malinche, the Aztec noblewoman who became the mistress of the explorer/conqueror Hernán Cortés, and then was abandoned by him when he returned to Spain. Her children were the first mestizos, making her the mythical mother of my race. This knowledge was both saddening and joyous because it made me more aware of all the pain that the mestizos had suffered at the hands of both the European conquerors and the indigenous people. Many of them were the children of rape, and they were truly a people in between both races, trying to find a life for themselves.

At this time, I began to live in two worlds. Monday through Friday, I was climbing the ladder of success in the professional world, moving up from staff nurse to head nurse of psychiatry to director of nursing at the local hospital. I was making it in the dominant, white, English-speaking culture, dressing the part and being the model health-care professional. Meanwhile, any chance I could get on holidays, weekends, or during vacation time, I would shed my Western clothes and put on my huaraches and my *huipiles*. I would head to Mexico, tie my ritual red bandana around my head, and live with the curanderos.

Eventually the tensions of moving between two such diametrically opposed realities created a cultural crisis. I wasn't sure anymore who I really was. Was I a modern Chicana, a professional woman who was highly successful in my chosen field—or was I a mestiza who had returned to her roots and was studying curanderismo? How did all of the pieces of my identity fit together?

One thing was certain, as my understanding of curanderismo grew, I became more and more dissatisfied with the things I saw happening around me in the hospitals where I worked. Once, when I was working as nurse manager of psychiatry in a teaching hospital, I tried to voice my concerns about a psychiatrist's decision to give electric shock treatment to one of the patients, a twenty-three-year-old manic-depressive. The doctor did not honor either the patient's pleas for help or my intuitive sense that "something bad was going to happen." He only wanted to hear clinical, rational facts. On the day of the patient's treatment, when I went to her room, she looked at me with eyes full of *justo*, begging me to intervene. I felt powerless. Sure enough, this woman died from a massive overdose of the anesthesia used in her treatment. Her cries for help went unheard because intuition is not honored in hospitals.

Another patient I cared for was a nineteen-year-old teen who had been told by a psychiatrist that if he kept on refusing to eat, the staff would insert a tube through his nose into his stomach to force-feed him. The young man was psychotic and kept saying that "voices" were telling him not to eat. When I took him his lunch tray, he begged me, "Please don't make me eat this food. Something terrible will happen." Again, my intuition told me that hospital intervention would be wrong for this patient, but the doctor was adamant. The young man was force-fed and, two hours later, he was found dead. He had hung himself with sheets he had tied together and hung over the shower stall.

It was becoming more and more clear to me that many of the so-called mentally ill people coming into the psychiatric hospital were really suffering from serious soul loss, and that none of the psychiatric treatments or shock treatments they were undergoing were doing them any good. It was as if I were watching a revolving door of patients being admitted, treated, and then released, only to return.

What I really longed to do was spend more time in Mexico, learning about and working with a medicine that made sense to me and got lasting results, yet I was still clinging to the idea that I needed to be a nurse and progress in my career. Finally I decided that, if I was going to stay in nursing, I would at least work in the best hospital I could find. I applied for a job at the prestigious Neuropsychiatric Institute at UCLA, was accepted, packed up my belongings and my two children, and moved to Los Angeles. One of the first and best things that I did when I moved there was to reclaim my lost name. Since no one knew me, I decided to become Elena again.

I felt very isolated while living in L.A. In that city's crowded, noisy environment, I missed the mountains of El Paso and felt that I was out of touch with nature. For the first time in my life, I was not able to pass over the Texas border and easily visit Mexico. Although there were other Chicanos in Los Angeles, few of them were living in the exclusive neighborhood where I was renting an apartment, and even fewer were working at the level that I was at the institute. Some of my colleagues, in fact, were quite open about the discomfort that they felt in working with, or under, a Chicana, and made thoughtlessly cruel remarks. For example, during one evaluation that I conducted, one of my staff members confessed that she was having problems taking orders from me because the only Mexicans she had ever been around were the maids.

On the plus side, I was acquiring valuable experience and knowledge working with the physically and emotionally abused children at the institute. I was learning more about the effects of medications on patients, what worked and what did not work. I also met many compassionate healers among the nurses, doctors, and staff. These individuals confirmed my belief that loving attention was often the best medicine that anyone could offer.

In spite of what I was learning at the institute, I finally decided that it was time to make a life change. There, just as with my other hospital jobs, no matter how much I wanted to use what I knew about curanderismo, there was little room for ceremonies, *pláticas,* and eagle feathers. I realized that the modern medical model that I had to follow as a nurse left out so much of what made up a human being—the soul, the client's spiritual beliefs, the complexity of human experience, and the need for personalized treatment. Realizing that what I had been searching for as a healer was not going to be found in psychiatric hospitals, no matter how good they were, I decided that it was time to get out of hospital work altogether. By now, my experiences had taught me that the techniques of curanderismo often worked where Western medicine failed—and worked more thoroughly and deeply where Western medicine succeeded.

But the question I had to answer next was, "Where do I go now and what do I do?" I felt that I couldn't just go back to El Paso because I had burned my bridges behind me. I had made the front page of the local newspaper with a "Nurse Goes a Long Way" headline, and the article had even stated that I was going to work on my Ph.D. in nursing (a misconception). My friends had thrown going-away parties for me and *despedidas,* traditional ceremonies for saying good-bye. After a year, I felt too uncomfortable to return home, as if I would be going backward and not forward if I did so.

Remembering the times I had spent in New Mexico, I decided that I would have a better chance to use my skills in a place where traditional healers were still respected. On my trips there to do ceremonies with Native Americans, I had fallen in love with the spirit of the land, with the sky and mountains that were always changing, moment by moment, as the light played upon them; with the ochers, reds, browns, and blacks of the mesas; with the fragrant, wild openness of the desert that teemed with animals and birds; with the streams that rushed down through the canyons in the mountains, or meandered past hot springs. I applied for a position as the director of the Albuquerque Rape Crisis Center and was hired.

After a year of isolation in Los Angeles, I was happy to be out of the city and back into a culture that I felt comfortable with. By then, I had also integrated my name, Elena, back into my soul. Once I settled in and began to feel relaxed again in my long skirts and huaraches, I started to do more ceremonies with the indigenous people of New Mexico, going deeper into my spiritual practice. One of the things I began to do was the "long dances," all-night dances for the winter solstice and all-day dances for the summer solstice. I also began to attend local sweat lodges and pipe ceremonies.

Participating in ceremonies with the Native Americans felt very comfortable, but I began to realize that what I really longed for was to belong to my own tribe. Chicanos in the United States have a cultural unity of a sort, but they have become detribalized. I wondered if it would be possible for me to return to Mexico and find a tribe from which my blood was descended and rejoin myself to a tradition. Shortly after that, I heard about a powerful curandero named Maestro Andres Segura who was willing to accept Chicanos into his tribe and to teach them his tradition. Maestro Segura was a *jefe* (chief) in the *Danza Azteca,* a powerful ceremonial tradition that has been passed on from parent to child for hundreds of years. At this time I knew I needed guidance, a place where my spirit could feel at home, and this sounded like an answer to my prayers. There was a group of Chicano *danzantes* in New Mexico who were going through the same experience I had gone through, wanting to get back to their indigenous roots. After I had attended one of their ceremonies, they invited me into a talking circle and I voiced my intent. When they asked me what my reasons were for wanting to join the tribe, I explained to them what I was going through. They told me what joining their tradition would entail, that I would have obligations that I had to fulfill, ceremonies I had to attend in Mexico, such as the ceremony on December 12 for the Virgin of Guadalupe, who represents for the Aztecs an ancient goddess. I would also have special duties and obligations in New Mexico, such the ceremony for the Día de los Muertos, the Day of the Dead. I prepared my *vestuario,* my sacred clothing for the ceremonies, and my headdress of feathers, and went with them on their next trip to Mexico.

There, in the early 1980s, I met Andres Segura for the first time. Maestro Segura was one of the keepers of indigenous wisdom who had been asked by his counsel of elders to make periodic visits to the United States as a teacher and emissary. These elders came from a tradition of guardians who for centuries had maintained the Mexihka (Aztec) traditions. As an elder of the Concheros (Aztec dance), he served as a bridge between indigenous peoples everywhere. Although he was in his mid-sixties when I met him, I was amazed at how vigorous he was. About five foot six, he had very long black flowing hair, and a body that was very solid and strong. His presence was so powerful that it was intimidating, and he had incredible dark piercing eyes that seemed to look right through me. Acutely aware of everything that was going on around him, he was very careful to make sure that things were done correctly. Once when the group was singing *alabanzas,* which is a type of chant, I wasn't singing because I didn't know the words. He came up to me and said, "Sing.

You learn the words by just opening your mouth and singing." When I told him that I was embarrassed about my voice (I sing out of tune), he said, "We are people. People sing." He helped me to open up my voice and have courage, and he didn't like to hear excuses.

When I went with his tribe to my first ceremony, a spring ceremony when the *danzantes* symbolically break the frozen earth to allow the new growth to come up, we didn't take anything modern with us to the sacred site. Instead of a camp stove, we took braziers, old-style stoves, to cook with. Getting ready to dance was an unforgettable experience. That particular *danza* lasted one day, proceeded by a *velación*, an all-night vigil. It takes all night to prepare the mind, soul, and spirit for the danza.

Getting dressed with the other dancers was also a beautiful experience. I had prepared my sacred clothes and my *penacho*, my sacred headdress, and learned the *danzas* from my compadres in New Mexico. I remember getting dressed, the magnificent colors, watching the men and women putting on their beautiful headdresses, the sounds of the rattles and the *oyoyotes*, the shells tied to their ankles. I was thinking, "Oh, here are my people and we are going out in ceremony together." When we walked out together to the sound of the *conchas*, it was as if my soul had been hovering around outside of me and had, all of a sudden, rushed back into my body. I felt as if I had finally come home. There was an incredible smell of copal in the air, and the sound of forty people all walking rhythmically in unison with their *oyoyotes*, shaking their rattles in unison, made me feel as if I could fly. *Danza* is very powerful, and sound and vibration are very powerful. My heart rejoiced to know that here was a tradition that was alive, intact, as it had been for five hundred years since it had gone underground at the time of the Conquest. Not one dance step had been changed.

Maestro Segura used to say, "Life is *danza, danza* is life. You dance as the universe dances." It's wonderful to go out and dance all night, pull out all the stops, and feel so good, but there is something so much more powerful in sacred dance. It takes years to learn the dances, so I didn't know them very well, but when you are dancing with a group of forty people who know those steps intimately, you just go with the group energy, and the next thing you know, you are dancing right along with them. Maestro Segura often said to me, "Your feet, your spirit, your heart, all of you knows the steps. Maybe your mind doesn't know them, but a part of you does. Let go. It's part of your genetic memory; it's all there. Remember also that you are not just men and women, you are warriors, dancing to maintain the tradition." In the *danzante,* the individual is really not who is doing the dancing, it's the community. You have to let go of your local self, and dance in your quantum self.

I loved watching the elders dance, those who were born into the *danza.* I was amazed at how much strength they had, and how they kept up with the younger people. They might not jump up into the air as much, but they were strong dancers. And unlike in the West, the children were not peripheral to the ceremony. They slept peacefully within the circle, nurtured by the drum that was like a great heartbeat.

I was also impressed with the sense of community I found. When the dancers went to buy the food for the ceremony, everyone contributed, even the poorest person. I was touched by the community's humility, the openness in every member's face and heart. They made me feel as if I were a long-lost relative. They gave me a sense of family and belonging.

To add icing to the cake, Maestro Andres Segura was also a powerful curandero who knew not just one part of the medicine but all of it. There were always a lot of children at the campsite during these danza ceremonies, which went on for days, and he taught me how to treat them for earaches, colic, dysentery, and *empacho* using herbs and different types of massage. He was very knowledgeable about herbology and was always pointing out herbs and their preparations, showing me how to gather and use the ones that grew in the area. He worked on the children and adults using pressure points, massage, and a technique that the Chinese refer to as *moxibustion* in which a long narrow tube is placed over one or more of the body's pressure points. A flame is held to the other end of the skinny tube, "warming up" the pressure point. Maestro Segura was very well known in Mexico City where he lived, and patients would come to see him for a wide variety of conditions. He also lectured throughout Mexico and the United States on Aztec cosmology. He was the first *curandero total* that I had ever met.

Maestro Segura also helped me to become a better counselor in my work in the U.S. When I told him about some of the women I was seeing at the Rape Crisis Center, he suggested ways to treat them for *susto*. One of these methods involved digging a hole in the earth, burying the woman with her head sticking out in the direction of the north, and letting the earth absorb her pain, ground her energy, and heal her. Sadly, I realized that I couldn't do that with the women at the center because policies and procedures bound me to only certain types of treatments. He also reminded me that, after a rape, a woman who was trying to resume sex with a partner would feel very vulnerable if her breasts were touched. He suggested that I counsel the husband to be very careful about touching his partner's breasts because she would need time to be comfortable with that touch again. Afterward, when I asked some of the women at the rape crisis center if this was how they felt, they said yes. Many admitted that they hadn't been able to let their partner touch their breasts since the rape.

My experiences in Mexico weren't always wonderful. There were plenty of times when I felt lost, inadequate, hungry, cold, and frustrated. I often went without sleep and food during all-night ceremonies, and I became ill with dysentery and parasites on many occasions. One particular incident that stands out in my mind was the time I was doing a five-day ceremony in a sacred site south of Mexico City. I had many duties. Not only did I have to dance from sunrise to sunset but, along with the other women, I had to make the breakfast and evening meal for the whole group. Because I was studying with Maestro Segura, I also had to learn how to take care of the children who were ill, which involved collecting and preparing herbs and learning more techniques of massage.

The group had set up camp at a graveyard, and the tent I was sleeping in was crowded with about thirty adults and children. All I had was a tiny space the size of my sleeping bag. On the third night I woke up in the middle of the night and realized that I had soiled myself. This was the most horrible thing that could have happened to me—my worst nightmare. Everybody else was asleep. Beginning to feel very nauseated, I went outside where it was raining lightly and steadily and began to wander around, not knowing what to do. In the darkness, I saw some huge rats. Terrified and feeling totally alone, I became violently ill, vomiting and having severe diarrhea. I did not know what to do, and felt great shame about my condition. I kept asking myself what I was doing out there in the middle of nowhere when I could have been home in New Mexico, safe in my bed.

Suddenly Maestro Segura appeared out of the darkness and asked me what I was doing. I told him that I was sick and that I had soiled myself. I started to cry and felt as if I were three years old. He was very harsh, and said, "What is wrong with you?"

At first I thought he meant, "What are you sick with?" and I answered by saying, "Well, my stomach hurts and I just threw up."

He said, "No, what is wrong with you?"

I didn't know what to answer, I felt so much shame. And then he told me, "Your community is inside that tent, your family. Most of us are healers. Were you going to wander around like an idiot all night long? Why didn't you ask for help?" At that moment, I realized that it had never occurred to me to ask for help because I had become so used to taking care of my own needs. This pattern had begun in childhood when I was not always properly taken care of by my parents, and had learned to mother myself. In the ensuing years, I had developed great pride in being independent. I realized that I really didn't know what it felt like to be a member of a community.

Maestro Segura took both my arms and applied acupressure to my forearms. The moment he did that, I burst out crying. It's as if he knew exactly where to touch me to release my pain. Then he took me inside the tent and woke up one of the women, and they helped me to change into clean clothes. After I was comfortable, they both gave me very loving healing, which included applying moxibustion to the pressure points on my forearms, ankles, and knees. Maestro Segura could be very harsh, but he could also be loving. He's been one of my greatest teachers so far.

The next day he relieved me of my duties, and told me how to prepare the teas to help with my diarrhea. I stayed back at the camp with some of the mothers who had young children and reflected on the fact that I had learned something profound. This had been a very harsh way to learn it, but I realized that perhaps it was the only way that I *could* learn in my life.

On another occasion, a friend and I planned to attend a ceremony for the Virgin of Guadalupe, and decided to drive all the way to Mexico from Albuquerque. When we stopped for a break in a small town in northern Mexico to visit the little plaza in the Zócalo, a bird shit all over my head. I turned to my friend and said jokingly, "I hope this is not an omen." Little did I know what lay ahead.

When I got to the site of the ceremony, Maestro Segura told me that I was going to be La Malinche, his counterpart, the female lead who carries the fire all during the ceremony. Petrified, I realized that I didn't feel prepared for such a complex responsibility. This proved to be the case. I had a very difficult time maintaining the fire, which was not supposed to go out during the entire two days of the ceremony, and I scorched my fingers several times. We danced all day with another tribe, had an all-night vigil, and then the next day danced at the Basilica, an old Spanish church built on an an-

cient Aztec sacred site. I made many mistakes, and each time
Maestro Segura's piercing eyes had told me that he was not
pleased with me. I could hardly wait until everything was
over. Again, I kept asking myself, "What am I doing here
when I could be home safe in New Mexico?"

After forty-eight hours of ceremony, which had left me
completely exhausted, the group was just about to finish.
While they were doing the last ritual to the five directions,
one of the compadres' capes got too close to the candle that
was part of the sacred altar. As he turned, the tassel on his
cape caught fire. I quickly leaned down and moved the candle. Just as quickly, the maestro stopped the ceremony and
was right on top of me, tremendously angry, looking at me
with his piercing eyes and shouting, "Why did you move the
candle?"

"Maestro," I said, "the compadre's cape was on fire."

"A three-year-old has more sense than you do. Don't you
know that your job is to protect the light? You never move
the light."

I was so exhausted and so confused that I lost my temper
and looked at my teacher with anger. When he saw that, he
said to me, "Nobody told you to be here. If you don't like it,
just get out right now."

This was a moment of truth for me. There was a very
strong part of me that wanted to do just that, just to run away.
I had to make a decision in half an instant, and I chose to stay.
I lowered my eyes to change the vibration of that energy I
was putting out to him, and said, "I'm sorry. Please forgive
me, Maestro."

We finished the ceremony and, afterward, he told me to
wait until he came for me. He left me standing at the ceremo-

nial site for an hour that seemed like an eternity, and I cried the entire time while Japanese and German tourists took pictures of me in my sacred clothing, holding my *sahumador* and weeping. It was one of the darkest moments of my life.

The next day while we were having breakfast, I asked maestro Segura why he had shouted at me like that. I had cried all night until my eyes were almost swollen shut. He said, "You had a very important job to do, to keep the light going for all of us. This is not performance dance. We are dancing to preserve the tradition. Before you moved the light, you could have pushed the compadre aside. Someone would have taken care of him. You have to think about the bigger picture." Then he looked at me, and said, "Will you ever move the candle again?"

I said, "No."

"Then I have done my job."

Ever since then, I have never moved the candle. When my clients come to do ceremony with me, and place their candles on the altar, I never move them. As difficult as that lesson was, I realized that I had always been taking care of other people's specific needs, never thinking in terms of the bigger picture. Now I had learned to do that. Something else in me had shifted, and I became more aware of what codependency really was.

Months later, I underwent a third major shift. Following another ceremony, in which the tribe had been dancing all day long, the people were all gathered together having dinner. One of the Mexican Indians turned to me, and asked, "What are you doing here? Why are you trying to be an Indian? You are a half-breed and a Yankee."

To me, it felt as if he had just thrown ice-cold water in my face. I looked at him shocked, and said, "What? A Yankee?"

He said, "Yes, you're from the U.S. You have everything you want over there. Most of you can't even speak Spanish."

At that point, I decided to open my heart to him and tell him what it was really like where I came from. "I'm not a Yankee, I'm a Chicana," I said. "I'm proud of my indigenous roots, and I'm proud to be here. In the U.S., they call us wetbacks and Mexicans, and tell us to go back where we came from because we don't belong there. We don't speak our language because it was taken away from us. As children, our parents and teachers spanked us when we spoke Spanish. The white culture told us that we were inferior. Now you are telling me that I am a Yankee. Then where do I belong?"

We ended up having a long discussion in which I educated him about Chicanos and their longing to feel connected to Mexico and their indigenous roots. I told him that I wanted to be in Mexico so that I could reclaim a lost part of myself, and that I had every right to be there. It was not my fault that I was a half-breed. We came to a very beautiful place of understanding, and he thanked me for educating him about my plight in the U.S. He had thought it was easy for us and didn't realize that Chicanos were discriminated against. He had thought we just didn't want to learn our traditions.

This conversation marked another major shift in my consciousness. I realized that I was not an Indian and not a white of European descent, but a mestiza. This was my destiny, this was what had happened to me, and I realized that I needed to be proud of who I was, of *all* the parts of myself.

For me this realization marked a major soul retrieval. I finally knew who I was and, from that point on, I started to change. It wasn't necessary to be dashing back to Mexico all the time, or to always wear *huipiles*. I realized that being an Indian was only part of my identity. I was a Chicana, born and raised in the U.S., bilingual and bicultural, and I was very grateful for all of the opportunities that I had received here. Although I still wore my indigenous clothing, I started to incorporate more variety into the way I dressed. I wore my professional clothes to work, then came home, took off my suits and put on my long skirts and *huipiles*. I also started to write more poetry and bilingual plays, reclaiming my *mesti-zaje* heritage. I realized that my people, the mestizos, are a bridge. They can live in both worlds. I didn't have to feel any-more that I didn't have a home because I did have one. My soul didn't have to fly off in different directions. It could stay inside of me now that I realized how beautiful it was to be a mestiza. I no longer felt ashamed, no longer felt as if I were the product of a bastard race of people.

My family could not help but notice a shift in me. Once while I was in El Paso visiting my kids, I walked in wearing a very smart suit. My son Abel stared at me in surprise, and said, "You're not an Indian anymore!?" He was completely serious. It was as if he were saying, "What are you now, Mom?" While I knew that this kind of experience is common among many women who get married in their teens and at some point need to go through their own stages of adult de-velopment, it reminded me of how guilty I had felt doing so. I knew that all of the dramatic transitions I had gone through on my journey must have been difficult for my children. Be-ing true to your need to find out who you are is very hard for women who have children early in life before they've had a chance to explore their identity.

Looking back over all the experiences of the last few decades, I realized that if I had had a grandmother or mother to teach me curanderismo and guide me through, everything would have been different. Instead I had to go back to Mexico like a brand-new baby. There I learned a lot of skills I didn't have—not all of them having to do with curanderismo. One time, when I was helping some other women to prepare dinner, my job was to prepare the carrots. I peeled them until they were shiny and clean, and cut a big chunk off the top and the bottom. When one of the women saw all the waste, she said, "You know, we are not from the United States and we don't waste the way you do. Look at all that food you are throwing away. We are too poor to waste anything here."

Experiences like this had made me feel inadequate and shameful, making me wonder what I was doing here. Many times I had entertained fantasies of coming back home to New Mexico, going to the mall and buying myself a lot of things, fixing myself a fancy dinner, and taking a long hot shower with lots of wasted water. I felt like Scarlett O'Hara, wanting to get out of there and never be hungry again. Sometimes it had all been too much, and I felt as if I couldn't stand another minute of being reminded of all the things I had that many of the people in Mexico didn't have. The people I shared ceremony with weren't just having a temporary experience of privation; this is how many of them lived every day. I didn't want to see any more poverty, any more mothers and babies begging on the streets of Mexico. I didn't want to see any outstretched hands. I just wanted to return to my cushy hospital job and wear my pumps and my panty hose and my silk blouses. At such times I asked myself, "Why do I want to do this? It's too hard, too painful, too sad."

Yet I realized, as I took stock and looked back over my life of the past twenty-two years, that all of the experiences I had gone through in Mexico and in the U.S. had been necessary for my training as a curandera—working at doctors' offices and in hospitals, visiting the curanderos who taught me so much, learning from my teachers in Mexico. I finally felt as if I had enough education to begin really practicing what I had learned.

My work in the doctors' offices had clearly shown me that my natural curiosity and intuition were leading me toward the nursing profession. There I received validation and encouragement from the nurses, who saw my talent and encouraged me to go to school and study. At the hospital in Los Angeles where I counseled physically, sexually, and emotionally abused children I learned about the harm that we can do to our young, and how severely we can damage them. The hearts of these kids were so broken, but as young as they were, and even after receiving so much abuse, it was amazing to me how strong their spirits still were. Many times the kids would end up in my lap, or I would be braiding a young girl's hair, and those moments would be more therapeutic than any medical procedure. Sometimes the kids would forget that I was there and just gather round and talk to each other, unselfconsciously. From those experiences, I learned that it can often be better just to listen to the kids instead of getting them into a private room and questioning them with a clipboard.

In the psychiatric hospitals where I worked as a nurse, I learned about many types of treatment modalities—family therapy, individual therapy—and what worked and what didn't. I didn't see much success with shock treatments and psychotropic drugs. What I found useful were heart-to-heart talks, a healthy diet, and art therapy. Sometimes I found it helpful to notice the small things, such as how my Chicano patients in the hospital missed familiar foods like rice and beans. It didn't take much effort to encourage the dietitian to be more aware of these preferences, and to provide these patients with foods that they found familiar and comforting.

Now I was ready to use what I had learned. I officially left the *danza* and began to think about what the next stage of my future as a healer might be.

Chapter Three

Tools and Ceremonies of a Curandera

I had hoped that things would be different when I began working at the Rape Crisis Center in Albuquerque, but trying to be a curandera as well as a psychiatric counselor was still difficult. The staff was uncomfortable when I tried to bring in my eagle feather, my copal, and my *sahumador* because they felt that I was imposing my religious beliefs on our clients. I even received criticism when I created a small altar in my office. I was especially surprised at the reaction from my two Chicana colleagues and my African-American colleague, who I thought would be supportive of my desire to honor my culture. They told me that if I wanted to bring my religion into the treatment room, then *all* religions had to be brought in. This mindset may have been politically correct, but it made it very hard to bring in *any* religions in a useful form.

I knew from experience that some of the techniques I had learned from Maestro Segura, such as burying in the earth a woman who had been raped in order to help her with her grounding, could be very effective, but, again, my co-workers were either frightened or uneasy about such an idea. It was too unorthodox for them. Nevertheless, the few times that I was able to do this with women were very healing. I would bury the woman in the earth, all but her head. Then I would stay with her throughout the experience, protecting her from being hurt, wiping away any insects that might come near her face, and reassuring her if she felt any panic. When a person has been so badly traumatized, being enveloped by the earth for a few hours is purifying and allows us to surrender our heaviness to the earth.

Other times at the center, I was able to sneak in aspects of curanderismo that seemed to fit within the parameters of established treatment modalities. For example, at that time anatomically correct dolls were being used by doctors and psychotherapists to teach children about good and bad touching. Since I didn't want my patients to have just an intellectual understanding of the soul but something that could help them to achieve a real transformation, I saw these dolls as a wonderful tool. In my counseling sessions, I used dolls to symbolize the part of the soul that was lost during a rape, or the part that had been sexually abused in childhood. I would ask a client to buy or make a doll that she felt symbolized that part of herself. Then, in a makeshift soul retrieval, I would hide the doll in my office and create a ceremony in which the woman looked for the lost or wounded part of herself, found it, and reintegrated it back into her being.

I was deeply moved by how this ceremony affected my patients, especially the incest survivors. Interacting with the dolls had a tremendous healing effect for them because it enabled them to reexperience and heal their trauma in a deep physical, emotional, and psychological way. When they found the hidden doll, they would hold it as if it were a real part of themselves, cradling it to their chests and kissing it. In reality, when they did this, they were loving themselves. They would talk to the dolls, their "soul" fragment, and tell it that the terrible things that had happened to them weren't their fault and that there was nothing wrong with them. Many rape victims do blame themselves. They often believe that if they just hadn't gone to that one particular bar, or worn that sexy outfit, or danced with that man, then they wouldn't have been raped. Now these women were able to stop punishing themselves for the terrible wrong that had been done to them.

Even though I was able to incorporate a few aspects of curanderismo into my work at the Rape Crisis Center, I ultimately had to acknowledge that the barriers to my bringing in the sacred severely restricted the depth of the healing work that I could do. It is unthinkable for a curandero not to call upon Divine Energy for help before he or she begins to work. Divine Energy was the very cornerstone and foundation of my healing work. It had never mattered to me *what* kind of belief system a client followed. Whether they were Christians, Buddhists, pantheists, Aztecs, or Jews, I could usually come up with something that was meaningful for them. And I never believed that I was the one doing the healing—it was Divine Energy working through both myself and my client.

With a great deal of nervousness, but an unshakable belief that I was doing the right thing, I decided that I had to turn in my resignation at the center and become a curandera full-time. For the first time in my life I was without a guaranteed weekly paycheck and benefits such as health insurance. Cashing in my retirement fund, I used the money to buy a home in Rio Rancho with a soul-inspiring view of the Sandia Mountains. I remodeled the garage into a treatment room, making it as comfortable as possible. I put in thick carpeting, soundproofing, an altar, a massage table, a comfortable couch on which to have my *pláticas*, and a place to store my files, drums, rattles, dolls, candles, and other objects that I used in my ceremonies. Now all that remained for me to do was to send out flyers. I had no idea if anyone would want to come and see this psychotherapist who had incorporated curanderismo into her work, but I was willing to give it a try. My soul demanded nothing less.

The response was better than anything I could possibly have hoped for. I was amazed at the kinds of people who came through my treatment room door. Rich people, poor people, people from Mexico, people from the pueblos who had no medicine man, *viejitas* (grandmothers) who were so happy that they could find someone to give them a *limpia*. I saw health-care professionals of all types—nurses, Ph.D. psychologists, and even a few doctors. People loved the effects of the therapy and would pass the word along to friends and family. Soon people were coming to see me from all over New Mexico.

Many of my clients offered me encouragement and validation, and that meant a great deal. One *viejita* I gave a *limpia* to started to get goosebumps. She gave me a blessing, and said, "I know that you are doing God's work, because when a person gets goosebumps, this is a proof that god's spirit has come into their body." Many Chicanos of my parents' generation would tell me that they had grown up with healers who did the same kinds of ceremonies that I did. Although they had gotten away from curanderismo for one reason or another, they were happy to have found that form of healing again. They'd say, "You are authentic, you are doing a good job." Hearing these words made me feel as if giving up all my security in the professional world had been worth it.

Sometimes I would see very traditional people from the reservations. I remember in particular one very beautiful eighty- or ninety-year-old Navajo woman. She hadn't been able to find a medicine man, and someone had told her about me, so she had asked one of her grandsons to bring her. She wore all of her traditional clothing, a long skirt, a crushed-velvet blouse, and a silver-and-turquoise belt. She was very pleased with her treatment and validated me by saying, "I felt so much at home. When you do smudgings, you do very much the same things that we do." I had given her a *limpia*, but her people called it a smudging. For me, it was such an honor to treat her that when she asked me how much she owed me, I didn't want to charge her. The woman insisted.

She opened up her white hankie, took out a five-dollar bill, and said, "No, this is for you." I put that five on my altar and left it there for many weeks, because I felt so blessed. I believe it brought me a lot of luck.

One of the things I had to figure out at the beginning of my practice was what to ask for my work. Many people feel that curanderos shouldn't charge because it is a sacred calling, and, at first, I really did try to make a living purely from donations, but it just didn't work out. A client would tell me about his $330-a-day cocaine habit, and then give me ten, fifteen, or twenty dollars for a session that had lasted an hour and a half. This showed me the value that people put on healing.

After struggling for a long, long time over this issue, I finally decided to charge a standard psychotherapist's fee with a sliding scale. I never turn away anyone who really needs my help, and I'm also willing to barter and try to work things out with people. But I also realize that I can't pay my mortgage in chickens. In the old days, all the needs of the curanderos were taken care of by the town. The villagers would provide them with food—chickens, eggs, fresh cow and deer meat—all of their firewood, and cloth so that they could clothe themselves. I still see remnants of this custom in some of my clients. Even though they pay my standard fee, they also bring me gifts of vegetables from their gardens, chiles from the famous fields of Soccoro, and apples from Mexico during harvest time.

One Native American woman, who needed several treatments and couldn't afford to pay for them, built me a beautiful breakfast bar inlaid with gorgeous handmade ceramic tiles depicting Indian legends. That counter has become a place where people gather in my house because they love the energy.

Sometimes bartering can have unexpected and even comic effects. One man in his early thirties dropped by one afternoon and begged to see me. His wife had just left him, he was depressed, and he was stuck raising his kids all by himself. He desperately needed help, but had no money. At that time my backyard was in bad shape, so I made a deal that he would weed it and clean it up. When he came back that afternoon, he brought his one-year-old and three-year-old with him and asked me to watch them while he worked. I had to change diapers, feed, and comfort the cranky baby who was on a crying jag. Meanwhile, the little girl was running around, asking for a cookie and making a mess of the house. I remember standing at the back door with the baby on my hip, watching the man take care of my yard, and thinking, "Is this a good deal or a bad deal?" In the end, however, I decided that it was fine because this man wanted and needed to get better. He really wanted to transcend his sadness.

When the Well Runs Dry

One of the most important things I learned as my practice as a curandera developed is that healers need healing too. Somehow we all have the impression that social workers, nurses, doctors, psychologists, and chiropractors can heal themselves. This is not true. Health-care professionals need outside intervention as much as anyone. Over the years, many people have come to label me as "the healer's healer" because I do a lot of workshops that teach healers to take care of themselves, and I receive many referrals of this nature.

Many doctors, nurses, and psychiatrists working in hospitals and institutions pick up the sadness and heaviness of the people they treat. They often call me asking for advice about how they can incorporate spirituality into their work, or how they can make a space to heal the incredibly sad experiences that they go through. Stress levels and levels of exhaustion are high with these individuals. Many nurses tell me, "I never have time for myself. I don't even have time to eat or to empty my bladder. I have so many patients to see, so many crises that, by the end of the day, I often haven't even found time to eat."

My daughter Sondie, a pediatric nurse, is a case in point. When babies die on her shift, she has to bathe the infant and assist the mother in saying good-bye. Her hospital provides a special place where the mother can sit in a rocking chair, hold her child, and take as much time as she needs to let it go. One evening my daughter called me and said, "Oh, mother, I am so sad. A woman lost her one-year-old baby today, and she wanted to hold him for hours. The staff wanted to take him to the funeral home, and I had to intervene on her behalf. I am so tired, what can I do?"

It kills the soul when doctors or nurses can't take the time to grieve and release their sadness, but our hospitals and institutions are not set up for that. Instead, health-care professionals are expected to stay objective and keep on going. The giving and emptying of oneself without being replenished creates a lot of burnout in the medical profession. You have a terrible day watching people suffer and die, and then, at the end of your shift, you are expected to sit down and calmly write up all your charts. You desperately want to leave *right now* and go home to your family for comfort, but you can't.

It is important for healers to learn how to take care of themselves. When I get bad news, for example, I smudge (cleanse) myself thoroughly with the smoke of sage or *copal*. I also cleanse my house often and give my healing room a periodic spiritual cleansing. I always give myself a *limpia* between clients, something that is very hard to do for health professionals, who go from patient to patient with no pauses in between. In my lectures, I always advise doctors, nurses, and psychotherapists to try to release the energy they accumulate in the course of their work, even if it means just taking a quick calming breath between patients. Ministering to so much pain and suffering, they run the risk of bringing some of that energy with them to the next patient if they don't take care of it. Even if they only have a few minutes, they can go to the bathroom and do a brief silent meditation or prayer. To keep this energy away from their homes and families, they can set up a simple altar with objects or pictures that have meaning to them, and smudge themselves in front of it when they get home from work at the end of the day.

I also ask other curanderas to give me *limpias*. My friends Flordemayo and Bernadette, my teacher Ehekateotl, my sister Irma, and my apprentices all give me *limpias*. On a regular basis I go to a natural stream and clean my eagle feathers and thank the Great Spirit for my tools. I clean my *sahumador* with dirt from the earth and thank Mother Earth. I follow what I preach, and I have found this to be extremely valuable in keeping myself healthy and my energy clear for the next patient.

Tools and Ceremonies

Altars

When I first set up my treatment room, I began with my altar. Why does a curandero need an altar? Because it acts as a focus for the sacred. After taking hundreds of injured or emotionally troubled people to my altar, I know how true this is. For me, my altar is the source of the divine energy that flows through me, giving me strength and insights into people's problems. The very first thing I do with new clients is to take them to my altar, where we pray together, asking God, in whatever form they imagine Him or Her to take, to help them to heal.

Traditionally a curandero's altar faces the east, the place of the rising sun, of new beginnings. Although there are certain traditional objects on the altar, such as representations of the four elements, each one reflects the unique personality of the person who creates it. One of the most striking things about my altar is the screen behind it, painted by my friend George Chacon. Each of its three panels is decorated with a beautiful painting of one aspect of female energy, and each of these images has profound meaning in my work.

On the left-hand panel is Coyolxauhqui, an Aztec goddess who used to be of the earth but is now a goddess of the sky. To the Aztecs, she represents the moon. Legend has it that the moon, along with her four hundred brothers, the stars, waged a battle against the great warrior Huitzilopochtli, the sun, to renew balance and harmony to the cosmos. This battle was waged on the hill of the serpent, where Huitzilopochtli killed her and dismembered her into five pieces. Coyolxauhqui became part of a constellation. Now, thanks to her, we can enjoy the equilibrium of day and night. She is the force that resides in the place between heaven and earth, and balances all that passes between these two places. With her left hand she transfers the divine energy born in the heart of heaven to human beings.

When I bring people, especially my women clients, to my altar, I point to Coyolxauhqui and say, "See, she is fragmented, just as we so often feel. She stands for the dualities, the light and the dark, that we all include within us." To me, Coyolxauhqui represents the idea that all women have more than one aspect to their nature. A woman has many names, takes on many roles, and often feels as if there are many different things happening inside of her all at once. We are not simple beings, we are complex. But this goddess can contain all of our dualities, no matter how much difficulty we have in reconciling them. She can help us embrace all of our paradoxes.

Pregnant, Coyolxauhqui is a symbol of creativity. All women are living embodiments of the creative force, and every woman understands the transformations of maternity, whether we are giving birth to flesh-and-blood children or to the children of our hearts—art, music, dance, painting, books. As we struggle in our personal battles, at times we all feel her *descoyuntada*—her dislocation and fatigue. But she also teaches us that when we go into battle, when we pass through the delivery of whatever we need to give birth to, we emerge transformed.

As a goddess dressed for battle, she teaches women how beautiful it is to reclaim their warriorship. Her names are: she who wears the mask of serpent rattles, the celestial dancer, universal mother, mother of dualities, and mother who glows in the dark. From this, I gave myself five names: daughter of dualities, raging abused little-girl me, two-headed serpent me, weird energy mine, and woman who glows in the dark. As women, we are always separating these aspects of the self, the mind, the body, the emotions, the spirit, and the soul. While it is true that these parts do have an essence, in reality, they are all one. Coyolxauhqui's nature as the mother of dualities is expressed in many ways: goddess who is both moon and constellation, day and night, male and female, war and peace, creation and giving, birth and sacrifice, the cyclical battle of night over day and day over night. All of us have these energies within, and Coyolxauhqui teaches us to recognize, heal, and balance them.

The middle panel of my altar bears an image of the Virgin of Guadalupe. To me, she represents two worlds coming together, the struggle of my people, the mestizos, to merge both Christian and Indian beliefs into one. I also see her as a symbol of heaven and earth combined. She is the Virgin Mary, feminine energy, the mediator who can take my clients' petitions straight to God. At the same time, she is Tonatzin, the Aztec earth goddess, who reminds us that we are part of the earth and should take care of her. The Virgin of Guadalupe wears a rope around her waist, which signifies to Indian people that she is pregnant. This is a beautiful reminder to us of new beginnings, of being pregnant with possibilities.

The right hand panel bears a painting of the new moon, which is a good time to start one's healing. Anytime you want to have a rebirth in your life, anytime that you have made up your mind to change, it is always good to do a ceremony during the new moon. The moon also represents female energy and, like the Virgin, she is a mediator.

On the altar itself, I have various images that represent the energies and forces that I call upon for help when I do healing work. Just as the female energy is represented by the images painted on the screen behind my altar, I also have images that embody male energy. One of the most important of these is the baby Jesus, and a cross that depicts Jesus' death. To me, Jesus was one of the greatest prophets who ever lived in this world. He lived among us as a poor man, he suffered as we did, and he died on the cross for us. I always tell my clients that, whatever our idea of God is, we are not supposed to suffer unnecessarily. Suffering is a part of life but, like anything else, it flows in and out of us. It is not supposed to become a permanent resident in our souls. People die, catastrophes happen, illnesses cause sadness, but when we come to a point of accepting what is and moving on, we can let go of unnecessary suffering.

Another important image on my altar is an Aztec warrior holding an eagle feather. Several elder curanderos have pointed out to me that they have actually seen this warrior standing next to me, and he is very much one of my protectors and spiritual guides.

I have a small stature of a Mayan Chacmool, which represents a rain god. I bought my Chacmool in Chichén Itzá the first time I went to Yucatan. To me, he represents my Mayan origins. He reclines on his back and elbows, his heels drawn up and his head raised and turned to the right, and holds an oval bowl on his stomach that is the perfect size for the egg that I use in my *limpias*. When I reach for the egg, I always see the rain god's face and know that he has transformed the egg's energy.

Even though I don't have a representation of the sun, which in my culture is a very potent male symbol, I always begin my ceremonies in the east, the place of the rising sun.

I always have fresh flowers on my altar because they attract positive energy and are also a part of the earth. When we have plants and flowers in our home, especially in our bedrooms, where we sleep and regenerate, they draw healing energy toward us.

The altar of every curandero includes objects that represent the four elements: earth, water, air, and fire. These elements teach us lessons about how to release toxins and harmful emotions from our bodies, and how to purify and ground ourselves. On my altar, stones, crystals, copal (incense), and charcoal represent earth. The earth is an organism like our own bodies, and must take in nourishment and release toxins just as we do. I tell my clients that we must ask the Creator to release us from the toxins of accumulated negative energy just as we release our bodily wastes through urination and defecation. When we do this, we return to our proper and balanced place within ourselves. The earth teaches us how to surrender our heaviness to her, rooting ourselves in the center of her gravity to obtain spiritual nourishment.

I always have a vessel filled with water on my altar to remind me and my clients that seas and the rivers are within us as well as outside of us—we are 75 percent water, and our bodily fluids nourish every cell in our bodies. Our arteries carry oxygenated blood to the heart, and our veins carry away the oxygen-depleted blood. We pray to the Creator for clear inner oceans to bring in nourishment and help us to release toxins. Because our emotions are "watery," this element reminds us to allow our feelings to flow. Like babies, who one moment are screaming and the next smiling and gurgling, we should not get too attached to our emotions.

Air, or wind, is symbolized on my altar by the eagle feather. Human beings cannot live more than three to four minutes without breathing. When we inhale, our lungs bring in life-sustaining oxygen, and when we exhale we blow out the waste of carbon dioxide. In my tradition, wind connects us to the sky, symbolizing our upward desire to join with God, with the life force of this immense universe we call home.

The lighted candles on my altar and the smoke from the copal I burn in my ceremonies represent fire. Human beings carry fire with them because their bodies must create heat and energy in order to sustain life, burning the food that we eat into calories that provide energy for our cells. Our bodies burn with fever when we are purifying ourselves from an illness, and we feel a pleasant heat flow through us when we feel passion and make love. We can either use fire for destruction or to create warmth, healing, and affection. The destructive fires of rage can destroy everything in our paths, but if we ask the Creator to assist us in using our fire to burn away our petty egos and our destructive patterns, fire can become the great purifier.

Saints and Candles

The types of candles on my altar are the same as those used by many people of the Catholic faith, the glass candles of different colors with pictures of the saints on them that you can buy in most supermarkets. These saints act as mediators between the petitioner and God. When I am ready to do a ceremony that culminates with a *limpia* or a soul retrieval, I always ask my clients to bring a specific type of candle to light and place upon the altar, depending on their problem. In the Hispanic tradition we believe that each saint was human once and learned something very profound in his or her walk upon this earth. For this reason, each saint has a special gift for us. For example, we can petition St. Anthony when we want to recover something we have lost. This could be anything from a favorite earring to losing one's soul. I often ask people to bring a St. Anthony candle when I am doing soul-retrieval work with them. St. Martin de Caballero is petitioned when someone needs to find work, or needs help with his or her business. This saint rides a horse and has a sword. Below him on the ground is the person he is rescuing. Santo Niño de Atoche, the baby Jesus, is the candle one burns when praying for the healing of children's illnesses and problems with children. La Vírgen de Guadalupe, the patron saint of Mexico, is one of the most popular candles that you will see on the people's altars there. Loved and honored throughout the world, she's believed to be closest to God and, because she is a woman and can look at things from the vantage of a feminine perspective, she has a special understanding of the problems of humankind. When someone needs a great favor, I suggest that they bring El Sagrado Corazón de Jesús, a candle with an image of the sacred heart of Jesús. I always tell my Catholic clients that Jesús is "the main man" and that when they are really in need, they should go straight to him. There's a saint for everyone and everything.

St. Jude is a saint that played an important role in my life last year. Sometimes called the "saint of impossible causes," he is the being that you petition if you really need a miracle. I always tell my clients that a lot of us don't ask for that kind of help but that, sometimes, we simply have to admit to ourselves that a miracle is what we really need, often our only hope. I'm not one to ask for miracles very often, but I remember a time when I really needed one. Once, while I was taking a shower, I found a hard growth on the back of my leg. When I showed it to my doctor, she said that I was just feeling the hardness of my leg muscle. A few months later, I went back to her because the growth was getting larger and larger, and I was starting to feel some tingling in my leg. That was the beginning of a very frightening time for me. My doctor referred me to four others who all felt that I had a cancerous tumor. The last doctor was an oncologist who suggested an MRI, a very expensive procedure. Although I didn't have medical insurance, I agreed to the procedure because I wanted to be sure of the diagnosis. Afterward, the doctor told me that, according to the MRI, it looked as if I had a very dangerous type of cancer known as lymphosarcoma, and that I needed to go into the hospital in two days and get a biopsy. He said to be prepared for chemotherapy and possible amputation.

During those two days while I put my affairs in order, I was terrified. What was worse, I felt as if my muscular and shapely legs, which had always been one of my strongest assets, had betrayed me. The night before I went into the hospital, I lit a St. Jude candle and asked God for a miracle. I told God that I very rarely asked for a miracle, because most of the time I was busy being an intermediary between Him and my patients, but that this time I desperately needed one for myself. I told Him that I did not want cancer, chemotherapy, or to have my leg amputated. The next day I had the biopsy and the lump turned out to be a fatty tumor that was deeply imbedded in the muscle and was putting pressure on my sciatic nerve.

I believe that God and St. Jude gave me my miracle. As a nurse, I had been able to read my MRI and I had seen that the tumor looked dark, not white like a fatty tumor. Five doctors had all said the same thing, that they had been sure that I had cancer. We should ask for miracles more often.

Pláticas

On a typical day, I have enough energy to see about three or four patients for one, two, or three hours at a time. There are some healers who claim that they see as many as sixty, but they only work with each person for about ten or fifteen minutes. For myself, I would rather take the time and energy to work very deeply with a few clients than see a great many. That's not to say that there haven't been days when, out of compassion, I haven't seen more people than I can handle. When I overextend myself like that, there is always a price to pay. If I can't take care of myself, and get the proper rest and nourishment between clients, then I begin to feel tired and spiritually diminished. My own light begins to go out. In my workshops and in my practice, I always encourage healers to see only as many people as they can honestly handle. Each healer has to find her own pace that is most comfortable for her.

I see all kinds of people with all kinds of needs, and I tailor my treatments to each individual, something I was not really free to do when I worked in the modern medical world. Sometimes I do dream work, art therapy, or trance journeying with my patients. Sometimes we use psychodrama, acting out the problems, making masks, or even cross-dressing to get in touch with the masculine or feminine parts of a patient that he or she is ignoring. Sometimes we do straight psychotherapy with a *limpia.* It all depends on the needs of the patient. If the person who comes to me is an incest survivor and has never had therapy, her needs will be different from someone who has just broken up with her boyfriend and needs a letting-go ceremony. Those who need long-term work usually receive several *pláticas, limpias,* and soul retrievals.

Pláticas are one of the most important tools that I use in my practice. It's not really accurate to translate this word as "psychotherapy." A *plática* is a deep heart-to-heart talk that continues in installments for as long as it needs to—hours, weeks, even months—until everything has been said. Depending upon how emotionally well adjusted a person is, we will usually do a series of *pláticas* and *limpias.* I always choose odd numbers for the *limpias,* such as three, six, or nine, because these odd numbers are a part of my tradition. Even though I've asked all of my teachers why we do it this way, and they all have their reasons, the truth is, it is simply always done this way.

I don't believe in doing one big cathartic treatment, but in finding the pace of healing and transformation that feels most comfortable to the client. With some people, I can clearly see that their souls are frightened and that I need to move slowly and take my time helping them to remove their self-protective masks. Other people who come to me have done a tremendous amount of work on themselves. All they need is a *plática* and a *limpia,* and they are on their way again. For these individuals, the work we do together is like a spiritual, emotional, and physical tune-up—a preventative medicine that keeps them strong so that accumulated grief and stress can't creep up on them and make them sick. They might have one treatment, and then come for another one two or three months down the road. I remember one woman who came to me after she had been in a car accident that had given her a slight case of whiplash. She told me, "I have a slight *susto*, but I don't want to let it build up. I want to take care of it right now." When we are basically healthy, we know when we need a boost to keep ourselves that way.

Some people get so excited about healing that they want to jump right into their problem and solve it all at once, before they are really ready. I remember one woman who came to me dressed in an expensive business suit who described herself as "a real problem solver at work." She had decided that she needed to work on her issues with her abusive father, and wanted to begin seeing me twice a week. I told her that my schedule was full, and that I couldn't possibly begin seeing her. When she begged me, I felt sorry for her and found a place to work her in. Three days later, on the afternoon of the appointment, I waited and waited but she didn't come. Fifteen minutes before the hour was over, she arrived. She said, "You won't believe this, but I got lost."

"How did you get lost?" I asked. "You were just here three days ago."

"I was driving on the freeway and, all of a sudden, I didn't know where I was. I felt as if I had passed the exit, so I turned around and headed back. The next thing I knew, I was back in Santa Fe. I just couldn't believe it."

There was no time for her *limpia*, because I had another

client following her. But I knew that the experience was valuable. I told her, "This is just perfect. You were in a big hurry to do this, but your soul was not ready. So your soul got you lost. You have to honor this." She looked incredibly flustered when I said that, but she had to admit that I was right. She agreed to slow down and take her healing at its own pace.

In the Aztec tradition, *pláticas* are the place where a curandera not only learns the client's story but also has an opportunity to educate. The curandera finds out which habits and ideas might be contributing to the patient's illness, and then helps the patient to identify what needs to be released or modified. When I do a *plática,* all five of my senses, including my intuition, are completely focused on the story I am hearing from a patient. It's as if the motion of my pen writing his or her words on paper becomes a conduit to the energy that the client is emitting. I always let people know in advance that I need to connect with them on this deep level. Because my heart is open and my mind is receptive, I can feel the patient's mental, physical, and emotional vibrations.

For me, the energetic vibration that a person is emitting as she tells her story is as important, or even more important, than what she is saying. Once when I was staying at a hotel in Mexico City, the *patrón,* the owner, asked me if I would do a *limpia* for one of his maids whom everyone felt was suffering from *envidia.* He told me that this woman flew into rages, and that she was upsetting other members of his staff. I had sensed a very sweet spirit in this woman, so I was puzzled that he had described her as so violent and angry. When I actually began her treatment, I discovered that there were many factors contributing to her fits of temper. Some were physical. She had a ringing in her ear that kept her from sleeping, and lumps in her right breast. I told her that she had to go to the doctor and get a mammogram, and that she definitely needed to get her ear taken care of. I realized that she was suffering from sleep deprivation, which was the major contributor to her outbursts.

One of the most revealing moments during the *plática* came when I discovered that she felt that she had no home. Since she had never married, she had spent the last thirty-five years of her life living in a room at the hotel where she worked in Mexico City, returning to her father's house only on rare occasions. When I asked her to repeat the words "I have no home" several times, she did so with no outward show of emotion. But the grief that came pouring out of her being on the energetic level was devastating. I could not give her a home, but Divine Energy came to my aid and showed me what would help her. I told her that her true home was in her heart, and that her body was its temple. I explained that, if we could find a home within, this was infinitely more important than any house made of stone or wood. I urged her once again to go to the doctor and have her health problems taken care of. Then I gave her a *limpia* with flowers. Some of her grief lifted and her spirit became lighter. She embraced me, blessed me, and thanked me for helping her.

A Practical Spirituality

Finding out about my clients' spiritual beliefs is an important part of the *plática*. As I ask them questions about every aspect of their lives, and take down a complete medical history, I always ask them if they believe in God or a higher power. I really don't care what form that belief takes, or even if a person goes to church every Sunday, as long as they believe in something greater than themselves. If a client is an atheist, then it is almost impossible for us to work together because spirituality is at the core of my healing work.

It is a different matter, however, when someone has become so wounded that he or she no longer has enough energy to believe in God. Some people have gone through so many traumatic experiences as children that they are carrying a generational inheritance of pain, suffering, and sadness. As children, many of these people used to pray desperately to God to save them, but never felt that He gave them any help. One of my clients, who had been sexually abused as a child, used to try to make deals with Jesus every night. "If you stop making this happen, I promise I'll be a good girl. I'll help my mother more." But Jesus didn't save her. She wanted to believe in a higher power, but she was too beaten down even to hope that God would hear her.

When I begin working with someone, I need to know whether or not she has enough energy to believe in something. If she doesn't and wishes she could, then I start from there, helping her to regenerate some kind of belief system. I once worked with a woman who was raised in the Mormon Church. She hated God because her father, who was prominent in the Church, had sexually abused her. I have heard stories from many women whose husbands have physically, sexually, or emotionally abused them. When they have gone to their priests for advice, they have received no help. Sometimes the priest tells them to forgive their husbands, or to try harder, and these women come away feeling even more guilty and worthless than before. All too often some of the priests are themselves sexual abusers. People have good reasons to be mistrustful of organized religion, and in my practice, my patients often need to work on reestablishing their faith in God, or the universe, or the Great Goddess, or whatever belief system has meaning for them.

I also feel that it is important to see if they are comfortable with my spiritual beliefs. On the first visit, I always take my clients to the altar and explain my symbols and saints to them. Because I see so many people from so many different religions and spiritual philosophies, I feel that this is important. If a person is not comfortable with my beliefs, which happens rarely, then we don't work together. There has to be a real honesty between us. If we need to discuss their misgivings about my spiritual belief system for an entire *plática*, then that's what we do. I do not mean to give the impression that I expect my clients to believe as I do. I have certainly worked with all kinds of people, Buddhists, Native Americans, Goddess worshippers, Mormons, Christians, and Jews. I only ask that they have some sort of spiritual belief system themselves, and feel comfortable enough with mine to work with me.

Sometimes when people come to me, they are in a mode of simple spiritual survival. They are trying to believe in God, but they must reject everything that seems inauthentic, pious, or goody-two-shoes. For that reason, the down-to-earth practicality of curanderismo appeals to them. A woman named Sara wrote to me after her first *limpia:* "I don't remember a lot of what you said but my body absorbed it. Sometimes I have tried to pray but the dear God blah, blah, blah, or Zen mindfulness seemed too remote, perhaps too clean for my current circumstances. I like the way you prayed, it seemed down and dirty, if you know what I mean."

I see curanderismo as a middle ground. The curandera is not like the modern-day priest or doctor with narrowly prescribed dos and don'ts about spirituality and healing. In the treatment room of the curandera, down-and-dirty healing can take place. Imagine a woman who has four children and would like to find a way not to have any more because she is at the end of her strength. A good Catholic, first she goes to her priest, who has no children himself and is not really in a place to understand her. She tells him, "I am exhausted. I am at my wits' end. My husband and I are fighting about this. What can I do?" The priest will tell her that God forbids the use of birth control, and that she must obey God. Then she goes to the doctor to get some help. He tells her, "What's wrong with you? You can't keep having a child every year. You are going to wear yourself out. You don't have enough energy or resources to provide love for that many children, or to give them all an education."

So where can this woman go to get real help? The curandera has always been there to hold the middle ground, to offer her practical, tangible advice — something that she can use to make her life better. The curandera can give the woman herbs to help prevent conception. She can educate the woman to be more sensitive to her fertility cycles and her body. She can invite the woman's husband in to talk things out and see if he and his wife can find a way to reconcile their religious beliefs with their everyday life. The curandera knows that life is not black-and-white. A good curandera can help us find middle ground in a culture where balance, reality, and enlightened compromise are not always a part of our support systems, and where doctors are often clinical and impersonal and priests preach that using birth control will cause someone to go to hell.

Setting the Stage for Trust and Openness

Many people have taboos about what they can share with their medical doctor, priest, or psychotherapist, because they fear that they will be judged and labeled. A curandera does not put judgments on people or force them into neat categories of diagnosis. For this reason, it is easier for many patients to tell a curandera things that they have never told to anybody else.

The most important ingredient in the *plática* is trust. There is an exchange that happens between my heart and the heart of my clients. As I listen to their stories, I soon find myself in an altered state. I always dress in my indigenous clothing to differentiate myself from the modern counselor or doctor in the white lab coat. The peaceful energy of my treatment room, the burning candles, the smell of the incense, and the images of the gods and goddesses on my altar all make it easier for people to know that they are in sacred space where it is safe to *desahogar*, to get everything out of their heart. The word *desahogar* literally means "undrowning." It is a way of speaking freely that clears *empacho* and unblocks the throat chakra so that toxic emotions can be released. If patients are too tense or fearful to tell their story, I stop the *plática* and give them a massage. Sometimes things that patients need to say will come to them in that relaxed state.

A *plática* does not necessarily have to take place in my

treatment room, or even in any one particular place. It's not always easy to talk to a stranger, and sometimes I intuitively know that a client will be more comfortable telling her story outside. I have had incredible sessions with clients while walking through the desert with them, or sitting with them outside on my patio looking at the Sandia Mountains. Being in peaceful natural surroundings often helps me to get clues about their troubles and helps them remember things. Sometimes I take clients up into the mountains and sit with them next to a stream—whatever it takes to get things flowing.

It's not unusual for someone to come to me thinking he knows what his problem is, only to find that he really hasn't thought it through yet. For example, someone might tell me, "I'm here because I want to put closure on a relationship," but he is so filled with hate, bitterness, and the need for revenge that he is unprepared for that final step. It is not enough to just take our hatred and bitterness to God. We must be willing to ask sincerely for help in forgiving and releasing. When it is time for us to do the ceremony where I take the person's story to God, it is important that both of us be clear about where he really stands, how he is willing to change, and what he really wants. *Pláticas* help clarify these issues.

One time I was working with a woman who said she wanted to let go of a relationship that had ended, but kept following her ex-boyfriend around and sending nasty letters to his new girlfriend. During our *pláticas*, she said that she still loved this man. I told her that her behavior meant she was still hanging on through hate, not love, and that she was making herself sick both physically and emotionally. When I asked her if she was willing to let go, she said, "I thought I'd come here and you'd do a simple ceremony to take all of these things away."

I said, "No, you must be willing to work for it." I explained to her that true letting go meant forgiving the past, and acknowledging the good of all that we had learned. Letting go of the past means allowing new birth to come forth. To do that, we must first acknowledge how each person in our past has been our teacher.

If someone is obsessively ruminating about her ex, if she is calling him up and insulting him every few days, then this is what she must take to God. She might pray, "God, help me to let go of all these emotions that are making me ill." I always tell my clients that healing begins with an acceptance of what is. Sometimes we just can't let go of emotions right away because we need time to work them through. I always ask someone, "How recent was the breakup?" You can't pull on a tender shoot to make it grow faster. It takes energy to grieve, and we must give our grieving the energy it needs. In the Chicano tradition, we believe that when we suffer a loss, we have to pass through *luto,* a full four seasons of grieving, allowing ourselves the expression of all the emotions that come with that grief. For some people, a year might be too long because it is honestly their nature to be finished with grieving earlier than that. Others might have to go the full year, remembering the Christmases they spent with their ex, how they shared the season together, the things they did and the life they had built. Of course, if a person only dated someone for two months, she obviously doesn't have to do this, but if someone has been married for twenty years, it's a different thing.

Sometimes we must accept the fact that our grief may never entirely go away. Once I worked with a woman who wanted to be released from the grief that she felt from the suicide of her twenty-year-old son. A doctor had given her an antidepressant but I pointed out to her that antidepressants are for depression, not for grieving. Through our *pláticas,* I already knew that her life had been in good shape before her son died. She had a good marriage and said she had been happy. Now she felt inconsolably sad. I told her that it was normal that she should feel this way, because losing a child is a devastating experience. She needed to realize that she would eventually feel better but that, on some level, she would take that wound to her grave.

After we had been working together for a few weeks, this woman had a dream. In it, her son appeared to her and told her that he had gotten drunk, had a fight with his girlfriend, and committed suicide on an impulse. He said that he was sorry he had hurt her. She told me that this dream had comforted her, but that she would always long to feel her son's touch, to see his smile. Nothing could ever bring that back.

Sometimes I am in awe of the magnitude of people's pain and suffering. In some cases I simply have to accept the fact that there is a limit to what I can do, that I just can't fix everything, that sometimes it is okay to leave things unfixed. It is always difficult to comfort the profound pain of people who have lost children. I remember one man who came to me after the loss of his two sons. They had both been in their twenties and had died one year apart, in automobile crashes. The man was of Italian descent. Because in his culture passing one's name, heritage, and flesh down to one's sons is so important, he not only grieved for his sons but for the fact that his male seed had died out with them. To him, the second kind of loss was just as profound as the first. When it came time to do the ceremony for his soul retrieval, he brought the ashes of his two sons with him and told me that he would never let go of those ashes. That was all he had left of his seed.

I have seen tremendous spiritual strength in the people who have come to me for help. These individuals have been some of my greatest teachers. I especially remember an elderly woman who came for counseling at the Rape Crisis Center. Even though she was an extremely religious person, I could not call in God because the center was a secular setting. The woman had been brutally raped, vaginally and rectally, and, to be honest, I was so overwhelmed by her case that I hardly knew where to begin. To establish some sort of rapport, we had a *plática*. I asked her where she was born and about her childhood, and she began telling me about all the animals she had grown up with. Suddenly, following my intuition, I shared with her that my beloved cat had died that morning and that my heart was broken. This is not something that psychotherapists are supposed to do, to bring in their own "stuff," but somehow it felt right. The woman was very compassionate and asked me if there was anything going on in my family. I told her I was in the process of separating from my boyfriend. My cat had left to roam the neighborhood. He always returned, but that morning he didn't. We found him a block away where he had been run over.

She said, "Aha, I know what happened. Pets love us very dearly. They sense everything that is going on with us. Your cat sacrificed his life for you. So that nothing bad would happen to you, your cat created a focus for you and your boyfriend to grieve together." I realized that she was right. My boyfriend and I had cried deeply at the death of our cat, Chaco, that we had found together up in Chaco Canyon and grown to love dearly. In a real sense, Chaco symbolized the death of our relationship. While we were grieving for him, we were able to begin grieving for our own relationship.

I was astonished. Here was this woman whom I was supposed to be helping to recover from a horrifying trauma, and she had ended up helping me. Sharing my story, however, established a powerful bond between us. She began to open up and, from the stories she told me about the way she had grown up, I helped her find solutions for what she was going through.

To her the most horrible thing that had happened to her was not being raped but being taken away from her community. After the incident, her daughter had packed up her mother's things and put her into a spare bedroom in her daughter's house. When this happened, the woman felt as if she had truly died. What she really needed to recover was to return to her own little apartment and her community, which wasn't what her family thought was best for her. I was able to be her advocate and talk her family into letting her return to her own home.

My nursing skills also came in handy in this situation. When I asked the daughter to take her mother to a doctor and get her blood pressure and diabetes checked, the daughter said, "But we just had her checked last month." I was able to explain to her that when a person suffers a trauma, these things change. Sure enough, both the woman's blood pressure and her blood sugar levels were dangerously high.

Doing *pláticas* and *limpias* with my clients is truly a process that each person takes at his or her own pace. As each session is completed, I see the layers of trauma, *susto*, illness, and other people's projections peeling off my patients' souls like the skin of an onion. More and more of the energy that doesn't belong to them falls away as levels of protection are built up. Problems are clarified, and spiritual strength begins to build. Eventually we reach the smooth, grounded center of their being. I am always careful not to label the energies we examine as good or bad because I don't believe there are such things as good and bad energy. What I say to my clients is, "I am going to assist you in getting rid of the energy that doesn't belong to you. I am going to assist you in becoming yourself."

Ritual: The Ceremony of the Five Directions

Once a person has gone through a series of *pláticas* and is clear about what he or she wants to ask God for, we are ready to take his or her prayers to the altar and do what is called the ceremony of the five directions. The client's intent might be to mourn for someone or something that has died, to let go of a past relationship, or to get back in touch with a lost part of him- or herself. I always ask my clients to be on a special diet for three days preceding the ceremony—no meat and no alcohol, just good foods from the earth, fresh vegetables and fruits. Eating only these foods changes the client's energy and makes it easier for us to work together. I always tell the client that he or she should be prepared to ingest spirit, not to expend a lot of energy digesting protein.

I also ask the client to bring symbolic items to put in the four directions of the sacred space we will create on the floor of my healing room. Sometimes I have the client put things in the fifth direction, sometimes not. These items might be pictures of herself, her ancestors, or something she has lost; pictures and memorabilia from vacations she took with her partner; a doll or dolls that represent some aspect of the lost part of her soul or her childhood. Some people get quite creative. One client, who had become allergic to most foods, brought in a full-course meal, including her favorite dessert. She wanted either to get well so that she could eat these foods again, or to let go of them if that was her destiny. I put her food in the east, the place of mystery and new beginnings, on a beautiful place mat with utensils and a nice cloth napkin.

People have brought the clothes they wore as children. One woman brought a bright yellow sundress that she wore as a three-year-old. When she "saw" how little she was when she was first sexually abused, she was able to forgive herself for her incest. Another woman brought her wedding dress because she wanted to release her marriage of twenty-five years. People have brought baby shoes, music boxes, the cremated ashes of their beloved dead, paintings or ceramics they have made. A woman who had lost her two grown children made a ceramic angel holding two hearts. Another woman brought in a big box full of used tissues! She had saved all the tissues she had used crying over the betrayal of a five-year relationship. We burned the tissues as part of the ceremony because she wanted to let go of La Llorona, the "Weeping Woman."

If the client doesn't bring in enough things, or feels as if something is missing, I have drawers full of objects that she can use in the ceremony as she sees fit. I ask her to bring a candle that, in some way, represents what she is asking for. The candle also represents the connection between matter (the wax) and spirit (the flame.)

We will use as an example a client named Sandra who was trying to work through the pain, grief, and loss of a love relationship. Because human beings are the embodiment of na-

ture, Sandra and I began by working with and honoring the
five directions. In each direction, I asked her to create a shape
or symbolic form made out of cornmeal or whatever else felt
right to her. The shape could be a heart, a triangle, a box, a
hand, a flower, etc. When that was finished, I asked her to
place the items she had brought for each direction within the
shapes she had made. I teach my clients that we always make
offerings in the directions because these are symbolic food for
the spirit world and the ancestors to enlist their help and to
honor and respect them. It is similar to visiting loving friends
and bringing them a gift. It also implies an exchange of energy. We offer them a gift, we ask for their help.

First Sandra placed items in the west, the place where
things die and can be transformed into new life. Then she put
symbolic objects in the north, the place of ancestral wisdom.
This direction represents the things that we have inherited
from all of the generations that have come before us, the
learning that is in our bones and in our genetic code. I always
ask my clients to place pictures or symbols of their ancestors
in the north. The south represents that part of us that is
young, curious, and intuitive. Our soul often contains a little
child who has suffered many soul losses. It holds the imprint
of ourselves at the various ages when we suffered traumas
and became stuck in our development. We may have within
us a three-year-old who was sexually abused, a six-year-old
who was beaten, a twelve-year-old who was in a car accident,
and so on. But I also ask my clients to bring pictures that remind them of happier times, a happy baby face, the innocence
or the big smile that they forgot they had in them. Sandra
placed pictures of herself at various ages in the south, the
place of the soul, the place within us that always looks at life

as if it were brand-new. The fifth direction is where we end up after we have said our prayers in the other four directions. I usually do not mark it.

I always begin the ceremony of the five directions in the east, the place of the new dawn and new beginnings. The east reminds us that no matter how bad a day, decade, or childhood has been, we can always heal and start living again. The east is also a place of mystery. It reminds us that we really don't know what's ahead of us. There is tremendous power in that realization, the power of possibility. Human beings always try to plan ahead, but our plans are illusory because we don't know the most important thing—when we are going to die. Even people who decide to take control of their lives by committing suicide often botch the attempt and wake up to find that they are still here; or, worse, a person discovers that jumping off the building didn't end his life but made him a paraplegic. It doesn't matter what we have planned for the years ahead. We could die half an hour from now, so I remind my clients to look toward the beauty of the east and to celebrate life because we never know how long its precious gift will be ours. Since the color white symbolizes new beginnings, in the east Sandra puts a white candle, white flowers, an amulet that was given to her, and several pictures of happy babies.

The whole purpose of setting up the directions and placing objects in them is to tell the client's story. What people bring to be put in the five directions always shows me how serious they are about their healing. If they have forgotten all their props and their candle, I know that they are not yet ready for the ceremony. In these cases, I will lovingly suggest that we have another *plática* so that they keep reflecting on their story.

Once Sandra had placed all of the objects she brought in the appropriate directions, I lit my *sahumador* and burned co- pal. On the altar, I had already placed fresh water that I would break the egg into after I had passed it over her body during her *limpia.* I gave her a pinch of cornmeal and we went out into the backyard together where I instructed her to offer the cornmeal to my *romero* plant and ask its permission to pick a branch for her *limpia.* The path that leads from my healing room to the *romero* marks out a significant journey. As we walked it together, we could smell the plants of the desert, see the Sandia Mountains, breathe in the fresh air, and feel our- selves close to the earth. Sometimes people cry as they walk that path. I create all of this beauty for people because so many men and women who come to me for help haven't had much beauty in their lives.

Then we were ready to say our prayers to the five direc- tions. There are no time limits for this ceremony. It takes as long as it has to take. I told Sandra to hold the *romero* branch and her candle. Before she prayed, I reminded her that everything she said, all her tears and words, would go into that candle that she is carrying with her. After we have en- tirely finished the ceremony, we will place that candle on my altar where it will stay lit for seven days while I keep vigil over it. I will notice how it burns and take care of it for her. Every time I see the candle I will remember the ceremony and the intent my client put into it, and I will also continue to pray for him or her.

We began in the east, where Sandra stated her intention. I invited her to talk to God throughout the ceremony in what- ever way felt most comfortable. I said my ancient pre- Columbian prayers and invoked Divine Energy. At this point in the ceremony, I no longer follow a set ritual; I channel the energy according to God's guidance, and help teach each individual some important lessons about him- or herself. Whatever happens each step of the way comes directly from my heart and will be very specific to the person I am working with. Even though the lessons each direction teaches remain consistent, the ceremony is never the same; it is very personalized. The lesson we learn in this direction is that if we look toward the east, we can remember that we made it through the dark night and that we can tune in to the energy of the rising sun and be thankful that we are still here.

In the east, I thanked God for my life, for my family's life, for my client standing to my right, and for her family. I thanked Him for the mysteries of life. I told Sandra that if we make it a habit to thank God every day for this new life, then miracles happen. When I felt that I had finished making my prayers in the east, I asked Sandra to say her own prayers from her heart, as if God were standing right there in front of her. At this time during the ceremony, if I feel a client dissociating while she prays, I bring her back, perhaps suggesting that she focus her attention on the image of the Virgin or on Jesus on my altar. Praying for oneself during this sacred ceremony can be so powerful. Often people have gotten so far away from spirituality and from God that they become overwhelmed. When they touch the sacred again, sometimes they weep or sink down onto the ground, the experience is so powerful. Some people have many things to say in the east, some people just say a few words, but I always guide them into talking from the heart, not the head. All of our prayers are said out loud.

Once Sandra had finished saying her prayers in the east,

then we journeyed to the west, the direction of the setting sun. This is the hardest direction for most people because it often represents the graveyard of their belief systems, their loved ones, and their relationships. It is hard for people to look at what they have decided to let go of, the marriage, the pictures, the beloved father or mother, the career, the child who has grown up and left the house. I always ask my clients to ask God's help in letting go of their feelings of sorrow, ego, self-importance, pity, fear, and hatred. Often I help release these things from their energy body with my hands.

Since I know that the west is so powerful, sometimes I just invite the client to sit down with me because I know it will take time. I picked up a picture of Sandra's ex-husband. "Tell tell me what he taught you. Tell me what you liked about him," I suggested. In this way, I allowed her to grieve fully the loss of this relationship, all the happy times they had spent together, raising their children, the wonderful vacation in Hawaii, the things they had shared, both happy and sorrowful. Sometimes in the west a person will be overcome with feelings of grief or anger, and I will encourage her to express these feelings as long and as loudly as she wants. *"Aiii, he betrayed me, he left me, the fucking asshole, but I can't let go of him,"* Sandra cried, weeping.

When all her emotions and sadness finally came out, I gave Sandra a chance to say good-bye. If she could, I encouraged her to say her farewells not in anger but in love, because I believe that that is the only way that we can truly let go of someone. Sandra was able to say, "Good-bye, I love you and I wish you well. I hope that your fondest dreams come true." When this happens, this is real healing.

Then we went to the north. In the north we find our

symbols of the past, our relics and our ancestors. Most people become very emotional in the north, calling out to a grandmother or another elder who loved and cared for them. I called in Sandra's *abuelitas* and *abuelitos*, her grandmothers and grandfathers, and encouraged her to talk to her ancestors and remember the past. This direction is powerful because many of us have had grandparents who have literally and figuratively saved our lives. If the west is the place where so much grieving, anger, pity, and self-importance comes out, the north is where most people find hope. The north has always been very meaningful to me, so much so that once I had a dream in which my ancestors came to me and said, *"Mijita, you are too comfortable in the north. You keep coming to us and you stay in this direction too long. We want you to know that we are always with you and that you don't need to invoke us so much. Move on to other directions and see what you can learn there."* In the north, we can become like little children again. I used my body to be sensitive to Sandra's energy, to channel it and to move it. I told her what I was doing and that we can learn to do this for ourselves, that all of us have the ability within to tap into that energy and heal ourselves.

In the south we find all of the little children inside of us who were hurt and lost. Here I remembered all the stories that Sandra had shared with me and I talked to her about them. I asked her if she had a nickname, an affectionate diminutive of a name that she liked. I find that many times my clients do not like their full given names because their parents used their full names when calling out to them in anger. My first name, Ada, is my mother's name, and because of the conflicts I've had with my mother, I've always had conflicts with that name. I've had to reconcile myself with that. When I found out that in Spanish, Ada means "fairy," I lost a lot of the pain I felt from my name. It's the same for many people.

Sandra told me that her grandparents always used to call her little Sandi, so for her I called out, in a very affectionate way, "Sandi, little Sandi, come back, my darling, come back, my little one. You don't have to hide anymore, come back, come back." As I always do when calling the soul, I used different pitches, different intensities, and different tones of voice.

At times, it is hard to get those lost child parts to return, because the adult's life is filled with stress and choices that have not always been for the best. When this happens, I help the client to make compromises with herself. In this case, I told Sandra's child part, "I know Sandra has been working too hard, but she has promised to take better care of herself. She will not work as hard, and she will be good to you and take you out to places where you can relax and enjoy yourself."

As we move through the five directions, my clients often begin sobbing in certain directions. Through the *pláticas* that we have done together, I have learned many intimate details of their lives, and can mirror this information back to them clearly to help the emotional barriers they have erected to melt away. When it was Sandra's turn to say her prayers in each of the directions, her energy had moved from her head to her heart and she could really connect with the energy of her neglected soul. At this point, I often witness people communicating with those lost parts of themselves in an incredible way. People will make promises to their souls, comfort them, and promise to take care of them. Sometimes there is no connection at all. Whatever type of energy they use when talking to a particular aspect of themselves becomes an incredible assessment tool for me, helping me to understand where their soul is. I often use this ceremony as a preparation for a client's soul retrieval.

The fifth direction, which we arrive at when we have made a complete circle and passed through the other four, symbolizes community. It reminds us that we do not live as an island, that we need each other. There is space for everything in this circle, what we know, what we don't know, all our contradictions and paradoxes. I reminded Sandra that the fifth direction symbolizes the universe, and that we are a little planet whirling through space in a cosmos of galaxies. Ethnicity, age, color of skin, gender—none of that matters. Everything belongs in the circle where we are all one, all connected. The circle teaches us to see the bigger picture. It is always moving and evolving.

After Sandra and I had visited all of the directions, symbolizing that we had passed through her entire life, I placed her candle, which contained the energy of her intent and all her tears and prayers, on the altar and lit it. Once the candle is lit, I do not move it. I then began to pray, starting with an ancient pre-Columbian ritual in which I call in the energies of God. This prayer, which is called "The Light Prayer," is a secret, and I cannot record it here. As I finish this prayer, the ritual is sealed.

At that point, I always ask my clients to lie down on the massage table. I took Sandra over and gently helped her to lie down and get comfortable. Sandra had been weeping quite a bit, so I got her a tissue and a wet washcloth. I felt that Sandra could benefit from some soothing music, so I put one of

Enya's CDs in my player and turned it on. I helped Sandra to relax her breathing, uncross her hands and arms, and to be in an open, receptive place. Then I gave her a *limpia*, rubbing the egg all over her body, front and back, starting from her head and moving down to her toes.

During the *limpia*, I picked up Sandra's energy, assessed her emotional state, and noted where the blocks were in her energy body. After I finished with the egg, I broke it, dropped it into a glass of water, and "read" it. Basically what I do at such times is to look at the relationship between the egg yolk, which symbolizes the individual, and the egg white, which represents the energy that does not belong to the client because she has just released it in the ceremony of the five directions.

Then I used my eagle feather to sweep Sandra from head to toes, helping her to release the mental energy that she needed to get rid of—intellectualizing, false belief systems, ruminating, and obsessing—and blocked spiritual energy, in other words, anything that was keeping her from spirit. When I use the eagle feather on a client, it breaks up those energies. Then I usually visualize sending all of that energy up to the heavens or down to the earth. Heaven and earth know how to transmute all of our garbage; we don't.

I also swept Sandra's body with the *romero*. The *romero* plant has a very strong smell, very pungent, clean, and earthy, and is excellent for grounding and bringing a person back down to earth. It's another tool that I use to pick up energy that does not belong to someone. When I was finished giving Sandra these *limpias*, I "tucked in" her aura with my hands. At this point, Sandra was in a very relaxed and altered state, and I asked her to stay lying down for at least ten to fifteen minutes. I always advise my clients to go home and rest or do something nice for themselves after this ceremony — take a bubble bath, listen to soft music, or take a walk in nature. It is important that they engage in activities that keep them grounded and relaxed, enabling them to hold on to that spiritual feeling and let things gel with them.

It has been eleven years since I left the Rape Crisis Center and finally "came out" as a full-time curandera. I now consider being labeled strange or different as a compliment. At this time in my career as a healer, I have participated in thousands of *pláticas, limpias,* and soul retrievals. My heart and my intuition have expanded as I have witnessed people from all walks of life healing themselves. Where others see hopelessness, I see miracles. I know how desperate, crazy, and out of balance people can get, but I also know how amazingly a person can transcend his or her illness or psychological wound.

Curanderismo has given me the freedom and sacred space to honor my path as a healer and to put all of my experiences to good use, and it has given me the freedom to honor each of my clients as a highly creative, emotional, spiritual, and unique soul. When we give our wounds to God we find the spiritual strength to live our lives and accept our destiny. When we realize that our souls and spirits need as much attention as our bodies, minds, and feelings, we experience supreme equilibrium. We are whole again. I have learned to honor my own soul by not denying who I am. I was born to be a curandera and a nurse. I am now a *partera,* a midwife, to many souls who have lost their way.

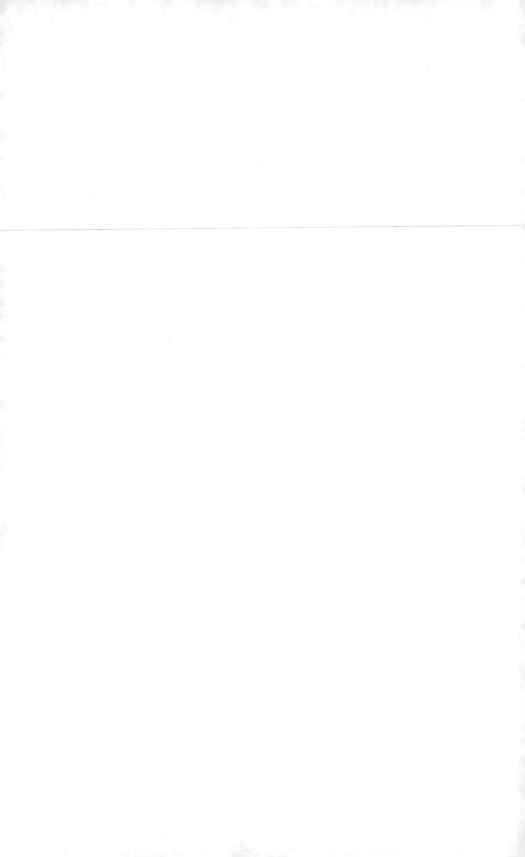

Chapter Four

The Weeping Soul

W hen I read books and articles written by sociologists and anthropologists on curanderismo, most of them refer to *susto* as a "folk disease" that only certain ethnic groups suffer from. As if every human being didn't have a soul! In my experience, the health of the soul and the spirit are at the basis of many physical and emotional ailments. The main reason I stopped working in structured institutions such as hospitals is not because my training as a nurse was not valuable to me.

169

It was because Western medicine does not incorporate the soul and spirit into the diagnosis and treatment of disease. Unless the needs of the soul can be addressed, there is a limit to what can be done for the body, mind, and emotions.

When I was working at UCLA with sexually abused children, the hospital was happy to have me lecture about curanderismo, but if I wanted to do a ritual or bring spirituality into a patient's care, they flatly refused to let me do so. Once I was working with an eight-year-old girl of Mexican descent who had been sexually abused by a neighbor. She would alternate between periods of uncontrollable rage and times when she would become almost catatonic, sitting in a corner and refusing to talk to anyone. When I had a meeting with her parents, they asked if it would be possible for me to do a soul retrieval for her. Their diagnosis of their child was that she had *susto*, which, of course, was true. The hospital's diagnosis was post-traumatic stress syndrome. When I approached the hospital about doing a soul retrieval as part of her treatment, they refused, calling it "an unknown medical treatment that might make the patient worse." They were afraid that it would "exacerbate a psychosis." This kind of situation has occurred over and over again in my nursing experience anytime I wanted to introduce some kind of spiritual or soul-oriented intervention in a hospital setting.

Only three times in my entire career as a nurse and curandera have medical doctors actually called me in to do a spiritual intervention. In each case, these doctors only asked for my help because they knew I had training in both curanderismo and Western medicine. One of these times I was called in to evaluate a man at the Santa Fe prison who was acting out in a violent and uncontrollable way. He had told the prison psychiatrist that he was *embrujado,* "bewitched," and the prison psychiatrist wanted to honor his cultural beliefs. As a curandera who was also a psychiatric nurse, I was the ideal person to interview him. As it turned out, the man was not cursed but suffering from paranoid schizophrenia. I listened to his problems and then gave him a *limpia.*

I have always believed that medical doctors and curanderos could benefit greatly from working closely with one another. My medical training has certainly made me aware of the signs of organic illness. If I notice that clients have a suspicious rash, or a lump in the breast, or signs of high blood pressure, I always strongly counsel them to go and visit their doctor. I also refer many of my clients to physicians for a complete medical examination or for lab work. If someone is already under the care of a medical doctor, I call up their physician and confer with him or her.

But there are times when a medical doctor cannot help people because Western medical practices traditionally exclude the soul and spirit. As the "science" of medicine has gone forward in this century, the care of the human has become very compartmentalized. The body goes to the doctor, the mind to the psychiatrist, and the soul and spirit to the church or synagogue. It is my belief that we cannot divide ourselves into pieces that way. If we want true and lasting wellness, we cannot leave the soul outside of the hospital and the doctor's office. I carry my soul and my spirituality with me everywhere I go, because I know that I am more than a body.

For example, if someone breaks her leg, it's not just the breaking of the bone but the *susto,* the soul loss that she suffers from, that has to be addressed. Many personal issues and vulnerabilities also arise in such situations. When the body's freedom is confined by a broken bone, the spirit longs for the mobility to do all the things that the person is used to doing. Simple, easy things such as walking, bathing, and getting dressed will become challenging tasks. A person might even begin to feel powerless because she now has to depend on a partner, family member, or friend to help her with her intimate needs. She will have to deal with feelings of powerlessness and fear, such as worries about missing work and paying expensive hospital bills. Depending upon the seriousness of the break, she will be in suspense as to how well her leg will function once the cast comes off, and how long it will take her to walk with ease. All elements of the personality are out of balance. Just putting a cast on her leg, and saying, "You'll be fine!" is not enough. The distress of the patient's soul and the pain of her emotional turmoil will not be lessened.

The Nature of the Spirit

A lot of people are confused about the difference between the soul and the spirit. Basically the spirit is the envelope that protects that soul from harm. If the spirit is relatively healthy, the soul will be too. How do we keep our spirit in good health? In the tradition taught to me by my Aztec teachers, the spirit is the part of us that is the sum total of our nutritional habits, whether good or bad; it is the energy generated from our feelings, whether balanced or unbalanced; and the energy created by our thoughts. The spirit is also the sum of our education and our intentions, and the part of our being that connects us to the "Great Spirit." A strong spirit buffers negative outside influences much as the skin of a fruit protects the fruit from decay and certain insects.

The condition of our spirit also affects our social relationships, whether other people are drawn to us in love and friendship or repelled by us. A spirit loaded with energy that does not belong to it becomes stagnant, heavy, and undesirable. When we cultivate unhealthy habits or remain stuck in unpleasant past events, our spirits can become musty and dried out. People do not want to be around these kinds of energies. If our spirits are light, healthy, and well balanced, vibrating to a frequency that resonates with universal Spirit, we attract and inspire others who are drawn to our energy and light. The way that we care for our spirit, and the life decisions that we make either consciously or unconsciously, are what determine whether we have a healthy or unhealthy relationship with self, family, community, and all living things.

An Aztec prayer that has great meaning for me ends in the words "so that we all might have light, peace, love, consciousness, and harmony." The sum total of these five elements—all in balance with one another—is what the Aztecs call "the fifth direction." Achieving harmony is a big factor in having a spirit that is strong and whole. The first ingredient for finding harmony is learning to love oneself—*all* of oneself. When we learn to love and accept even the shadow parts of ourselves, the parts we judge and criticize, we can then learn to love all living things. If we are in harmony with ourselves, we can even have a harmonious relationship with the bacteria in our bodies, promoting greater physical health.

Since the soul is dynamic and evolving, it needs the energy

of an intact spirit to propel it toward its potential. To heal the spirit and keep it strong, and to achieve harmony, we need to work toward becoming fully conscious. This means taking responsibility for our thoughts and actions, and working to heal our wounds so that we can remember ourselves and see the bigger picture. Doing these things helps to create a light spirit that can more easily find its way to divine Spirit because it can actually *see* God's light and be drawn toward it.

A Leg to Stand On

Whether or not our souls can recover from the traumatic things that happen to us has a lot to do with whether or not our spirit is functioning in a healthy, protective way. If we have a strong spirit, we can work through our difficulties, survive our hardships with a certain amount of grace, and bounce back again.

This truth can be seen in the lives of two men I treated who were both greatly wounded by their inability to stand and walk on strong legs. Back in the early eighties, long before I became a full-time curandera, I met a remarkable man named Ruben and his wife, Rosa. This couple had been high school sweethearts and were deeply in love. Ruben was a handsome Chicano with an outgoing personality, and Rosa was a dark attractive Chicana who was devoted to her two children. Ruben had received his Vietnam draft notice shortly after high school graduation, and they had wed before he shipped out.

I met this couple while I was the manager of a psychiatric

unit at a teaching hospital. We had a nurse's station marked by a wall that came up to about chest level, and Ruben enjoyed shocking me by "standing tall" in front of the station and asking for his pain medication. The reason this always startled me (my office was behind the station) was that I knew that he couldn't possibly be standing there. Both his legs were amputated above the knee! He had lost them in Vietnam while saving several of his buddies. Ruben got a tremendous kick out of supporting himself on the station with his powerful upper torso, making him look, from my vantage point, as if he had legs.

Ruben hated his wheelchair, but most of all he hated his injured body. Before his injury, for which he had been awarded the Congressional Medal of Honor, he had been over six feet tall and athletic. He had loved to play football and basketball, and had especially enjoyed running barefoot on sandy beaches along the coast of California where he and Rosa had grown up. He was a popular, handsome man with a big heart, but his injury had taken its toll on his spirit. He had become addicted to pain pills, alcohol, and pot, and had attempted suicide twice.

My heart went out to Ruben. I worked hard to help him with his addictions and suicidal tendencies, and I established a strong bond with both him and his wife. An extraordinary woman, Rosa truly loved her husband, just as he was, and had stood by him through his ups and downs. Sometimes, however, things were very hard for the two of them. For this reason, I also tried to help them through marital counseling. As much as Ruben loved his wife and kids, he told me that his soul had died in Vietnam. Without his strong athletic legs, it was hard for him to feel that he was a man anymore. He'd had numerous admissions to the local veteran's hospital and the psychiatric unit of the hospital where I worked, but what we had to offer did not seem to help him. What really needed healing was Ruben's broken spirit, but there was no understanding of or place for that kind of treatment in modern medicine. I knew this, and did the best I could within the confines of the hospital policy I was committed to obey, but I feared that my efforts were just not enough.

One night at home as I was preparing for bed, I got a call from Rosa. Crying so hard that I could barely understand her, she told me that Ruben had committed suicide that afternoon by shooting himself in the head with a shotgun. Rosa begged me for a *limpia*. She had heard me lecture on curanderismo and was desperate to find a way to cope with the intense pain of her sorrow. I did not know where she had gotten my home phone number, and it was against all hospital rules for me to see her, but I could not bear to leave her choking on her grief. I gave her directions to my home.

When she arrived, I could hardly believe the condition she was in. She smelled of pot and was so drunk she could barely walk straight. Her grief was so desperate, I didn't know what to do with her. I was also feeling my own *susto* at Ruben's death. I kept seeing him at the nurses' station, standing tall and supporting himself on his elbows, pretending he had legs to stand on. I could not believe that this robust man was gone.

Feeling completely lost, I asked Rosa to sit down facing me while I prayed for divine intervention. I asked her to close her eyes and take a few deep breaths. I burned copal and surrounded her with the healing smoke. I closed my own eyes, held her hands, and began to speak. "You knew and loved

Ruben more than anyone, Rosa! Tell me, what is he doing now?"

Tears ran down her cheeks and a smile spread across her face. "He is running! *El cabrón* is running!"

"Where is he?" I asked her. I knew that she was clearly seeing him in her mind's eye. "He is home," she whispered, "on the beach. I can see his footprints in the sand. He is loving the sensation of his feet hitting the sand. He is free, running as fast as his legs can take him."

I held Rosa as she poured out her grief, silently thanking the Creator for his presence and guidance. We both knew that Ruben was in a better place. It saddened me that Ruben's spirit had not been strong enough to protect his soul from being eaten away by the sorrow of losing his legs and his ability to walk, run, and stand tall. But I knew that Rosa would eventually heal because she loved her husband enough to let him go.

Mike, however, was a different story. A fifty-two-year-old Chicano, Mike came to see me recently requesting a *limpia* because he had been laid off from work and had not found a new job. Linda, his wife of thirty-four years, came with him. This couple had a strong and loving relationship and were devoted to each other and their children. After putting in thirty-two years at the bank he had worked for, Mike had been laid off due to downsizing. He could not collect his pension until he reached fifty-five years of age.

The rejection Mike was facing on his hunt for a new job brought up old feelings of anger and rejection. Mike had gotten polio when he was six months old and was unable to walk until he was five. He remembered getting around by dragging his left foot and holding on to furniture. When he was seven, he went through two years of treatments to stimulate his weak leg muscles that consisted of the doctor applying electric shock to his injured leg twice a day. These treatments were extremely painful and he hated them. Meanwhile he had to wear a brace in order to support his weak and atrophied leg. The kids in school made fun of him, mimicking his limp, and to this day Mike goes into a rage if he hears the word *cojo* (crippled). "Rejection became my worst enemy," Mike told me. "And I got into many fights. If people made fun of me, I would attack them and had to be pried off because I went in for the kill."

Mike had many surgeries and spent a large portion of his childhood in the state hospital for crippled children. Many of the surgeries he received there were experimental, and his average hospital stay for each was three months. He was isolated from his family during much of this time because the hospital was several hundred miles away from his home in Tucumcari, New Mexico. "I remember the first time I was hospitalized," he told me. "I did not see my mom for two weeks and couldn't stop crying because of the pain and loneliness. The nurses told me that only babies cried, and that if I did not stop, I would be placed in the 'dark room.' I learned to cry alone, and I grew up angry." Mike had to wear special high-top black shoes and an awkward heavy brace until he was twenty-one years old.

"Fitting in" became crucial to Mike. He would walk two miles to school on crutches so that he could walk along with his friends. When the coach refused to let him play on the baseball team, he became the batboy. Mike learned to play saxophone so that he could join the school band, but felt humiliated when the band director would not allow him to march with the rest of the kids because he could not keep up. He could only play at concerts and in the stadium at football games.

Mike told me that suiting up for physical education was the hardest thing he ever had to do. When he took off his clothes, he could not hide his crippled leg from his schoolmates in the locker room. He compensated for this weakness by exercising to make his upper torso very strong. No matter how hard he tried, however, he couldn't even begin to keep up with normal physical activities. One time in gym class he insisted on going up a rope with the rest of the boys only to realize, several feet off the ground, that he could not come down. Another time he hopped a freight train with his friends and realized that he had to jump off onto his weak legs. He broke his brace in the process. He felt "normal" when he went swimming, but it was humiliating to get out of the pool and drag himself, holding on to the wall, to his brace.

He didn't date very much, but when he did, he tried to impress the girls by being exceptionally well dressed. He spit-shined his ugly shoes until he could see his reflection, made sure his shirts and even his blue jeans were crisply starched.

In his teenaged years, he had many more painful surgeries, which included an operation on his good leg. Since his bad leg could not keep up with the growth in his good leg, the doctors decided to perform a procedure on the good leg to stop the bone from growing. This caused Mike to end up being shorter than he normally would have been. At this time in his life, he started using alcohol and pain pills as an escape from his pain.

Mike met Linda when he was twenty and she nineteen. "She was the best thing that ever happened to me," he said.

"She made me feel lovable and she still does. I have always wanted to give her the stars." They had raised three daughters together and considered themselves blessed and happy until Mike got laid off.

The rejection that Mike was experiencing was taking its toll on his spirit. On one visit he told me, "I have applied at sixty places and been rejected at every one. I can't help but feel that the reason I am being rejected is because of my disability. All the old feelings that I thought I had taken care of are coming back." Even though Linda and his family were very supportive of him, he was terrified that he would end up dependent on his wife. Between his unemployment insurance, the income from her full-time job, and the money Mike was making playing in a band on the weekends, they were making it, but just barely. For Mike, this was just not enough. He was being made anxious and physically sick by the feeling that they would be struggling to make ends meet for the rest of their lives.

Inside of Mike was a weeping soul that had never really been allowed to grieve. During our last visit together I worked on the repeated soul losses Mike had experienced from his frequent hospitalizations, his chronic pain, the mockery he had suffered from his peers, and the self-hate he felt for his *cojo* soul, the shadow side of his self. Remembering Ruben, I asked the Creator to help me to cocreate the healing that Mike needed.

I pointed out to Mike that, with his fifty-second birthday, he had just finished what the Aztecs call "the first cycle of life." I felt that he faced a choice at this point. He could either give in and give up, or he could stop looking at life as a bitter challenge, heal and bury the past, and choose a new life. I gently suggested that one of the reasons he was having so much trouble finding new work was that he was still feeling so much fear and hatred from his past. I also suggested that perhaps he was looking for work in the wrong place and needed to step back and reevaluate what he really wanted.

When I told him and Linda the story of Ruben, they were deeply moved. Mike identified with Ruben, and told me, "I always wanted to be a soldier and stand among a group of warriors, but I guess I've fought and won battles in my own way. I know that my experimental surgeries helped other people with similar problems. In fact, my beloved mother is recovering from an amazing procedure that might not have been possible without the research done on people like myself. Her hands were crippled with arthritis, and now her fingers are straight and beautiful. Kids like me were the experiments that taught the docs about muscles, ligaments, and bones."

Because of the work we had done together, the *pláticas*, *limpias*, and soul retrievals, Mike's spirit had gained strength and clarity. By coming to me willingly, ready to see his new "face and heart," he had made a choice to live. Ruben's spirit had been shattered in Vietnam along with his legs. He hobbled along with a crippled spirit until the drugs and alcohol had finally killed the fragments of soul that remained in his heart. Mike chose another way and was now ready for his next fifty-two years of life. He remembered his weeping soul and released the fear and hate from his spirit. Now both of his legs are standing on solid ground. Recently I was overjoyed to receive a message from Mike detailing his happiness at finally finding a job as the assistant manager of a bank.

Not all of us will go through the kind of debilitating experiences that Ruben and Mike went through, but being human means that, inevitably, there will be times in our life when we do get sick or experience traumatic events. If we are conscientiously willing to heal, care for, and preserve our spirit, most of the time we will find the strength within to bounce back from adversity.

Characteristics of the Soul

Whereas the spirit is energetic in nature and acts primarily as a protective shield and conduit between us and God, other people, and the living world, the soul is that part of us that includes all that we are: our talents, our hopes and dreams, our true voice, our nature, and our identity. Because all souls are unique, each person's soul is his or her spiritual fingerprint. The soul is the seat of creativity. It does not just sit there unchanging, but is always in the process of evolving, wanting to finish one stage of development and go on to the next.

In my tradition, we do not believe that the soul is somewhere out in space, ephemeral and holy. To us, it is very earthy, concrete, and embodied. This is very different from the picture offered by Western Christianity. At some point in our history, spirituality and medicine went their separate ways, and the soul went with one camp and the body with the other. I believe that it is time to reconcile this split. Curanderismo is a medicine that brings all parts of the human being into the healing equation.

In curanderismo, the most important thing about the soul is that it is sacred. A curandero will never touch the essence of a person's soul, never impose his or her own ideas upon it, because the soul should never be contaminated by another person's perceptions, projections, or opinions. In my tradition, we believe that when the soul is violated to such a degree that we cease to be who we truly are, the body may still live on but the soul is dead. In essence, that person no longer exists. We can see many examples of these "walking dead" in Western culture. The recent rash of teens going on killing sprees, murdering their parents and fellow students, is a good example of this. Many of these teenagers have suffered such severe childhood abuse to their souls that they have no sense of identity or hope. A soul cannot evolve under a climate of hopelessness.

There are many ways that the soul can be violated. During childhood, many people experience the slow chipping away of their desires and their individuality by subtle parental criticism. When parents force their own dreams and ambitions upon a child, trying to live through him or her, that is a form of soul murder.

Many people have experienced this form of soul violation. They live for years, never knowing that a big part of them has been denied. Then one day they wake up and don't know who they are anymore because they have spent years living for someone else. They cry and feel empty, but they don't know why. Angela, a woman in her mid-thirties, came to see me because of marital problems. Without realizing it, she had spent her entire married life always putting her husband and child's needs ahead of her own. This continually weakened her sense of identity and self-worth. As the years went by she had become obsessed with her appearance. Because she felt so insecure and self-conscious about how she looked, she was constantly changing the style and color of her hair. If she gained five pounds, she took laxatives and threw up. Anytime she was invited to a social event, she would spend hours trying on different outfits, trying to find the right look for the evening. The idea of having to please a roomful of people scared her to death. Would So-and-so criticize her because she was too sexy, too dumpy, or too fashion conscious? Since she had no sense of self, everyone else's opinions had to define her, and she would agonize over how she could present herself so that she would be accepted by everyone. When she looked in the mirror, which she did obsessively, she always saw a stranger.

Like many women in our culture who obsess about their weight or appearance, Angela's soul was dying to be noticed, to be found. Unconsciously she knew that she needed help, but she didn't know how to ask for it. Instead she used physical complaints to cry out for the love that she wasn't getting. If she felt a pain, she would hope that she needed surgery because then people would pay attention to her. If she got a stomachache, she wished for stomach cancer, because that meant that she would be nurtured and taken care of. What she was really trying to say when she complained of all these ailments was, "My soul is injured and needs help."

People often complain of or even actually develop physical problems to call attention to the needs of their soul. I had one client who had been sexually abused at an early age and had never been able to tell anyone about it. As a child, she used to fall on her knees all the time. When she ran to her parents and teachers with bloodied knees, they would try to figure out what was wrong with her. Were her ankles weak? Was she growing too fast and experiencing clumsiness because of growing pains?

Later, as an adult, this woman realized that she had really been calling out for help. At that age, she didn't know how to say, "Please help me, my soul has been injured." All she could do was to show people her bloodied knees. This was the physical manifestation of her wounded soul. She had no words for the fact that she had been raped but her soul knew that she needed love, understanding, and healing.

In my culture, we have always known that the soul can be injured as deeply as the body, mind, and emotions. We call this kind of wounding *susto*. Literally translated, this means "fright of the soul." Because the soul is sacred and should never be touched, when it is violated by traumatic experiences, it runs and hides, as if it had become frozen in time because of terrible events. We might not be able to say, "I was sexually abused at the age of three," but we might spend our entire childhood falling down on our bloody knees as a way of saying, "Look, something horrible happened to me."

Aspects of ourselves, such as whether we can sing, shout, or speak with our full voice, are other examples of the physical manifestations of soul loss. One woman told me about how, when she was six years old, a rapist had come up behind her and grabbed her by the throat. As he choked her and then raped her, she thought she was going to die. From that point on, she could only speak in a small, whispery, nonforceful voice. Her ability to connect herself to the world through speaking and to express emotions such as anger and pain through the voice, was taken from her. When she tried to get her children to behave, nothing would come out of her mouth but a pitiful little whine.

When I worked with her, one of the things I concentrated on was getting the woman to reclaim her ability to speak loudly. While she drew pictures, I would tell her to make certain types of sounds to help her release her voice. This was very hard for her. Then one day at home when her children were being particularly bad, she heard herself say "Stop that!" loudly and forcefully. She couldn't believe this was *she* talking. From that point on, her ability to speak improved more and more.

Soul loss can happen at any time, as we live through the traumas and shocks of our lives, and experience the violation and denial of our nature. Even if you are a person to whom nothing very dramatic has ever happened, you are not exempt from soul loss. Every one of us has, at one time or another, lost a part of our soul because of the cultural values we have all been forced to embrace. This loss might have happened in our parents' home, in school, during our first dating experiences, in college, at our jobs, or in our marriages. While some people can cope fairly well with these small *sustos* without really losing themselves, others who are extremely sensitive experience them as more wounding experiences.

One of the stories that I tell frequently in my workshops illustrates how we begin to lose parts of ourselves in childhood. Martita is a little girl of three who doesn't know yet that the trees and the earth can't really talk. She wakes up one morning and hears the birds singing to her. She hears the trees saying, "Come out and play with us." Full of joy, she leaps out of bed, gets dressed, and goes out into the backyard. There she finds a tiny bird that has fallen out of its nest. She picks it up and holds it in her palm, feeling its warm breast resting against her hand, and the life flowing through it. At that moment, she knows that she is one with all nature, with all life.

She also learns another lesson: that she is large. When she looks to her parents, she sees giants who pick her up in their arms, hold her, and care for her; but to this tiny bird, she is a giant too. There are some things in the world that she is larger than, and this understanding makes her feel expansive. When the bird opens its tiny mouth, she realizes that it is hungry. She puts it back down onto the ground and runs into the house, calling "Mommy, Mommy, I found a little bird in the backyard. I held it in my hand and it told me it was hungry. What should I do?"

Instead of helping her to feed the bird, the mother's face becomes angry and she yells, "What? You touched a bird? Martita! Don't you know that birds carry diseases? Don't ever touch an animal like that again. Go up to your room, right now."

The little girl goes to her room and cries. Suddenly something that was so beautiful, so mysterious, and made her feel so whole, has been taken from her. When she thinks of the bird, its warm little heart beating against the palm of her hand, she sees her mother's large angry face. Because she loves and needs her mother, and cannot survive without her, she cleans up her room and then draws her mother a beautiful picture. She goes downstairs and hands it to her mother, saying, "Look what I made for you, Mommy." The mother looks at the picture. "*Good* girl," she says. "And did you clean up your room?" "Yes, Mommy," the little girl says. "*Good* girl," repeats the mother.

Martita hears the messages behind what her mother is saying, and she learns what good girls do and do not do. She draws a beautiful picture for her father. "*Good* girl," he says when he sees it. When she goes to school, she tells her teacher that she will stay after class and do an extra homework assignment. "*Good* girl," the teacher says. Soon the little girl has figured out that being a good girl means pleasing others, so she goes through life trying to do that. But a part of her soul has been lost in the process, a part of who she really is and what she feels.

One day when she is walking down the street with her school friends, one of them sees a little bird that has fallen out of the nest and is calling for help. She starts to go over to investigate, and little Martita stops her. "Don't touch that bird! Birds have terrible diseases!" The joy she felt as part of nature has been replaced by fear. Her natural reactions to the helpless, warm, living bird have been replaced by a repugnance that goes against her whole being, but is nevertheless a part of her now. A piece of her ability to react to life spontaneously, with an open heart, has been suppressed. She doesn't dare respond that way, and she doesn't remember why or when it happened.

The Need for Accepting All Parts of Ourselves

To be whole, we have to be in touch with all parts of our nature. We go to the curandero to help us identify those lost parts of our souls and call them back. A curandero helps us to ask ourselves, "What sort of person am I? Am I earthy, quiet and soft, dramatic, extroverted, introverted, sensitive, stoic, artistic, analytical, intellectual, passionately emotional?" There are no right answers because there is no "right" kind of person to be. What is important is that we experience *all* the aspects of who we are.

It is very easy for us to judge ourselves harshly because we have all internalized a lifetime of judgments placed upon us by our parents, teachers, and significant others. For example, for many years I really had to struggle with the issue of being a sensitive person because my natural physical and emotional sensitivity had always gotten me into trouble as a child. If my mother forced me to eat my much-hated bowl of Cream of Wheat for breakfast, I would throw it up all over the table. This upset everyone. If I was out playing and got all dirty, I got a beating. I was so sensitive that I could not be consoled and would cry for hours. What really hurt me during such times was when my mother would say, *"Lágrimas de cocodrilo,"* "You are crying crocodile tears." Soon I began to hate the sensitive parts of me.

If an artistic child grows up in a family where it is not okay to be artistic and make a mess, not all right to color outside the lines or paint the sky green, the constant criticism soon becomes too much for the child, and she gives up certain parts of herself. In circumstances like this, there can be no safe expression of those aspects of her soul. As a child, I turned away from my dramatic, poetic side because that was the part that reminded me of my mother. She was so dramatic, passionate, and self-centered that I never wanted to be like her. It used to drive me crazy that she could never tell a story without embellishing it. To me these embellishments were embarrassing lies. He emotional mood swings scared me so much that I became frightened of deep emotions. My mother used to be in plays when she was a child, and she often spoke about how much pleasure they gave her. That made me afraid to be dramatic. When she committed suicide right before my college graduation, she even wrote a suicide note in a poem to each of her children. So whenever poems began to come to me, I would turn away from them because that energy frightened me. I became like little Martita, turning away in fear from the things that came spontaneously from my soul.

Once I was able to reclaim that lost part of my soul, the poems poured out and I began to act in plays. The passionate, beautiful, dramatic woman that I really was emerged and my true nature could be more purely expressed. I came to realize that without that part of my soul, there is a big part of Elena missing. This is the part that tells stories in my workshops, the part that creates psychodrama and ceremony so that my patients can be healed. This is the part that enables me to take a client into the bathroom, dress her up as a man, stand her in front of a mirror, and shock her into seeing and reclaiming the masculine part of herself.

What Is a Soul Retrieval?

Although workshops on soul retrievals have become a big draw on the New Age circuit, reclaiming these lost parts of oneself has been an important part of my culture for thousands of years. This practice is very, very old, and very useful. When we say that a soul is "lost," "runs away," or "hides," we are using a metaphor. According to my teacher Eheka- teotl, if our soul truly leaves our body, we die. What we really mean is that the part of our souls that went through injury, vi- olation, or trauma has become repressed. In the example above, what little Martita kept with her throughout her later life was a fear of birds. What she repressed was a sense of lost freedom, of being able to spread her wings and express her powerful feelings of knowing she was one with all of nature.

If this little girl were to come to me many years later as an adult, I would begin by giving her as many *pláticas* as were necessary to find out what parts of her being had been re- pressed. Then, if possible, I would take her to the location where she had originally had the experience. Perhaps we would go to that place in her backyard where she had first be- come aware of the power of her body and her oneness with nature, and I would show her how good and beautiful those feelings were. I would tell her, "Look at the sky, at the green- ness of the earth, feel the wind on your face, feel the power of the earth's energy flowing through you. Now imagine your- self holding that tiny bird in the palm of your hand, and feel the life in it." I would call out her name several times, asking that part of her soul to come back to her, and say, "See, you have done nothing wrong. It's good to feel the earth in your body, it's good to feel the life of the hurt bird pulsing through your fingers, and natural and good to have a desire to help it and feed it. See the sun, it is so beautiful and warm shining down on you, bathing your skin in well-being. There was never anything wrong with feeling the way you did. It was other people who filled you with fear, who shocked your ten- der, wide-open heart into hiding. Now, Martita, come back and feel the tremendous power of this moment, of your total unity with nature and the largeness of your soul."

Whether done at the scene of the loss, or in the safety of my treatment room, soul retrieval is a literal re-membering of ourselves. Through this process, we gently warm up those aspects of us that were frozen at the moment of the trauma of loss, and reunite with them. We call back the parts of us that were jarred into hiding, and allow them to return.

Facilitating a soul retrieval is something like being a detective. As I talk to my clients, I am always on the lookout for behaviors that seem normal to them but are clearly not normal. A hysterical fear of birds is not natural, so I would know where to look for Martita's trauma so that, together, we could begin to heal it.

Once a woman came to see me because she was having trouble with her marriage. During the *plática* I discovered that she always douched and took a very long shower after having sex with her husband. She was especially careful to scrub her private parts thoroughly. At the time, she was completely unaware that these were not things that everyone did following intercourse. When I asked her husband to come in and talk with us, he expressed a terrible sadness that his wife reacted this way. He missed the intimacy that comes after lovemaking, the holding and kissing, and the spooning together of two bodies before going to sleep. His wife's behavior made him feel very hurt and abandoned, and he wondered if there was something wrong with him that made her have to run into the bathroom and wash herself off.

After working with this woman for a long time, I discovered that she had been raped when she was a little girl. For years she had successfully repressed this memory, but the smell of semen coming from between her legs after she made love with her husband threatened to revive it. Her best defense was to rush into the shower and get rid of the smell.

She and I were able to go back in time and find, comfort, and heal that terrified little girl she had once been. We were able to help the woman she was now to begin to feel more comfortable with the natural smells of her husband's body.

A Soul Retrieval Can Be a Cultural Healing

Often a soul retrieval can result in people being reunited in a healthy way with their ethnic roots. For five years I worked with a woman named Donna who came to see me after her counselor, who was treating her at a psychiatric hospital following a suicide attempt, terminated her therapy. The reason the counselor gave for ending the therapy was that she was beginning to feel suffocated by Donna, as well as overresponsible for her. Donna claimed that she had not been trying to commit suicide but had been sleepwalking in the middle of a nightmare. She was dreaming that a pair of menacing hands were coming toward her. When she woke up, she was standing in her kitchen with a knife in her hands and blood all over her arm.

One of the first things Donna told me was that she had relationship addictions. Once she became involved with someone, she was haunted by fears of abandonment and insecurity. When a lover would have to go away for the weekend, she would plead with him not to leave her because she couldn't face the terror of being alone. Of course, this stifling need to cling to and smother people scared away many relationships.

Donna had been adopted when she was a year old, and knew nothing about her birth parents. She had been born in New Mexico but did not know where. Raised in a small town in the southern part of the state, she had moved to Albuquerque when she was twenty-one years old. She had never felt close to her adoptive mother, who was a very cold person who only touched Donna when it was absolutely necessary. Even though her father was warmer and more affectionate, Donna was afraid to let him in because his job required that he travel a lot and he was not home very much.

As a child Donna had suffered from various health problems such as a thyroid condition, chronic ear and bladder infections, and bed wetting. I felt that a lot of her physical problems had stemmed from the anxiety that she felt around her adopted mother. She had always felt like an outsider around the other children in the neighborhood, who left her out of their games and sports, and seldom invited her to their parties. She once told me that she used to swallow pennies because she knew that money had value and she wanted to be worth something.

Donna had so many other problems that it took us a long time to get to her adoption issues. Since she had been painfully raped in her early twenties, we decided that the first thing we had to do was to work on her rape issues and her low self-esteem. She also needed to grieve deeply the loss of her last relationship and the sad parting she'd had with her previous therapist. Because of her severe abandonment issues, it was important for me to establish a strong bond with her. Donna's insecurity often made that difficult. After disclosing something to me about herself, she would frequently say, "You're not going to leave me, are you?" Once, when we had reached a certain point in her therapy, she explained that she was terrified because this was the point where her last counselor had dropped her. She was terrified that I would do the same.

After Donna had made sufficient progress in all of these areas, I felt that it was time for us to take a look at what had happened to her during the first year of her life. When I brought up the possibility of looking for her birth parents, she was petrified. I told her I was suggesting this route because it would be difficult for me to do a really complete soul retrieval without knowing something about her first year. Nevertheless, when I saw Donna's fear, I decided to let the issue go for the time being. It is never a good idea to push someone into taking a step that he or she is not ready for. The *limpias* that we did were very healing for Donna and eventually helped her to find the spiritual strength and confidence to start the search for her birth parents.

Creating a stronger sense of self-love was a very important step toward Donna's soul retrieval. I often ask clients to find a doll that symbolizes their soul because this gives them a point of focus, a tool that can mirror parts of themselves that need nurturing and love. When the time was right, I asked Donna to find such a doll. The search for this doll was very painful for her because it caused a lot of old trauma to surface. At one point, she told me that she was feeling moments of panic, as if she were running out of time in her search. There was so much anxiety surrounding her task that, when she finally found the right doll and took it home, she had a difficult time getting it out of the box. The doll, which looked a lot like Donna, especially around the eyes, was beautiful, a tiny newborn with tightly clenched fists. Donna named it Ember, and we used it for a long time to help Donna to learn how to bond with herself. Because she knew nothing about self-bonding, she clung desperately to other people.

Donna told me that the only thing she knew about her birth mother was that she was forty-three years old when she gave birth and had been very ambivalent about whether or not she wanted to keep her child. For the first year of her life, Donna had been kept in limbo in a foster home, waiting for her mother's decision. Even as an adult, when Donna heard a baby cry, she would feel a pain in her chest.

I explained to Donna that she gave her spirit away to the people she became involved with because she was so hungry to be loved. She had not received the necessary bonding with her mother at birth, and she had gotten inadequate nurturing during her first year of life in the foster home. When she dialogued with her doll, it said to her, "I want to be loved and accepted. I was shut off from love."

One of the stories her adoptive mother had told her about her childhood was how she often threw up her food as a baby. When Donna did this, her adoptive mother would throw the food back at her. How terrifying this must have been for a small child. I was concerned at how matter-of-factly Donna told this story, without any feelings at all. Following a gut instinct that she needed to connect with this memory emotionally, I stood up, got some baby food out of the kitchen, and began forcibly shoving it into her mouth. Although she looked terrified, she passively accepted this behavior, only saying "Stop, stop," in a voice that was weak and shaky. I encouraged her to hit the palms of my hands and to say these words louder and more forcefully.

While this was going on, Donna had a memory recall of the event her adoptive mother had described. Through this, she was finally able to connect with and experience the rage and sadness she had felt as a small child, and to become more forceful and protective of herself. I reminded her that people will push you around and abuse you if you aren't in touch with your own sense of self-worth.

I did many ceremonies and *limpias* with Donna to help her let go of her painful relationships with her boyfriend and her previous counselor. After that, we were ready to begin a series of soul retrievals. In the early soul retrievals I took Donna on trance journeys to look for those lost parts of herself. She always came back from these journeys crying, stating that she had seen nothing, absolutely nothing, and that she was beginning to believe that she really didn't have a soul. She would see people and animals, and see herself doing certain things in the spirit world, but she would never find the lost soul she was seeking.

Finally she decided that she had enough courage to begin searching for her birth mother and the story of her early life. She was very scared. I promised that I would help her and went with her to a meeting of an organization called Operation Identify. This experience was very moving for me. I eventually became a volunteer with this organization and helped many other adoptees to find their biological mothers. OI did a search and found Donna's adoption records, and I agreed to be the liaison between Donna and her adoptive mother. If her biological mother refused to see her, however, I was not permitted to tell Donna anything about her history. I even had to sign a legal document promising this.

OI gave me the last address they had for her birth mother, a small town in New Mexico. I knocked on the door and told the woman who answered it who I was searching for. Looking very surprised, she said, "She died two years ago." I remember going to my car and just sitting there, taking deep breaths, and wondering how I was ever going to tell Donna that we had reached a dead end.

She took the news very hard, but the death of her birth mother had one unforeseen benefit: it gave Donna access to all her records. She brought them over to my house so that we could look through them together. To her great surprise, she found out that she was a full-blooded Hispanic. It took her a long time to absorb this information because she was light skinned and light haired and both her adoptive parents were Anglo.

We discovered that the woman who had answered the door was actually her mother's sister. When I got back in touch with the aunt, she told me that Donna had many living relatives. When these relatives heard about Donna, they all wanted to meet her. Because she was terrified at confronting her long-lost family, Donna begged me to go with her to give her courage. This experience was very healing for her. Donna's birth family prepared a delicious meal of enchiladas, sopaipillas, beans, and rice—all foods much beloved in Hispanic culture. They also showed her pictures of her relatives, allowing Donna to discover that she had "Uncle Chico's nose" and "Aunt Norah's mouth." Although it took several more months for her to work through the issues that arose as she began to integrate herself into her Hispanic culture, she felt peace that she had found her roots at last.

She also found out more about her birth parents. Her biological father, who had lived only a block away from her mom, had also died, which saddened her. The most powerful thing that she learned was that her mother had named her Juanita. When she learned her birth name, she felt as if she were going through an identity crisis, as if something had been forced on her that felt strange, alien, and disorienting.

The Day That Donna Found Her Soul

Now that Donna and I had all this information about the first year of her life, we felt ready to try another soul-retrieval ceremony. For this ceremony, I created a circle of blue cornmeal in my healing room with an opening that led to the altar. I put all of my sacred tools into that circle and sat down inside of it. With Donna's permission, I had already taken her doll, Ember, wrapped her in a little blanket, and hidden her in the east, the place of new beginnings. Ember's hiding place was in between the outer door of my treatment room and the iron security grating that locked in front of it.

I instructed Donna that, during this journey, she was to look for Ember and call her by name. I said that I would not be able to assist her unless she came through the opening into the cornmeal circle, sat down across from me, and asked for my help. I felt that this was important because Donna often got lost in her hopelessness. She was used to standing by passively while other people did the work for her. I wanted her to take the initiative to look for the doll herself, to decide if and when she needed help, and to actively take the step of asking for it.

For over an hour she called for Ember, looking for her everywhere—under the cushions on my couch, behind my bookshelves, in the drawers of the big dresser where I store my ritual items. Gradually, her cries became weaker and she began to stop, sit, and stare into space for long moments at a time. I had already told her that Ember was in that room, and that I was not tricking her. It hurt me to see her suffering like this, but I knew that I couldn't help her or say a word unless she asked. She had to help herself. All I could do was to sit still in the center of the cornmeal circle and send her my loving energy to reassure her and give her strength. As time passed, my bladder began to get full and I started to wonder how long I was going to have to sit there. I began to send her silent, desperate messages: "Donna, come ask for help. Donna, come ask for help."

Finally she did. She made that very important journey from the outside of the cornmeal circle to the inside where I was seated. She sat down across from me and looked at me with the saddest face. Looking about three years old, she said, "See, I don't have a soul." I instantly felt divine intervention flow through me. It was not I who spoke, it was the Creator. I said, "Call her Juanita." Looking straight into my eyes, she said, "Juanita," and then turned her head to the left, got up, and went straight to the door. When she opened it, there was her doll. Her face was pure ecstasy. She ran into the circle again and we both sobbed while I held her and her Juanita. I blew that soul essence into her crown chakra, and said, "Welcome home." Later she told me that when she thought of her soul, she had always felt as if she had left it on a doorstep somewhere, like an abandoned child. After the soul retrieval, she was able to tell that tiny doll, "Ember, you really do have a mother."

Donna is an example of a person who had experienced multiple *sustos*. She was abandoned by her mother as a child, separated from a foster mother that she had bonded with pending her adoption, adopted by a cold and abusive mother, often sick as a child, and raped at twenty. Yet she was able to heal beautifully. The last time I saw her she was in a loving relationship, had gotten a master's degree, and was working at a new job where she felt fulfilled. She was fully present in her body, and she was happy. Even though Donna had many problems when she first came to me, she worked hard and followed all of my suggestions. For example, when I suggested that she go see a *sobadora*, she did so. Because of her biological mother's ambivalence, she had not received adequate touch during her first year of life. She needed to learn how to nurture herself, and working with a *sobadora*, who gives nonsexual healing touch, was very good for her. She also went to music therapy to help her to find her voice. I knew that her soul was a singing soul and that her throat chakra needed to open up. Donna was truly committed to healing herself, and willing to take responsibility for her life and reclaim it.

The Power of Names

A crucial point that Donna's soul retrieval shows us is the importance of names. The identity of our soul is intimately tied to our names. In Malidoma Somé's culture in West Africa, the shaman asks a child its name while it is still in the mother's womb. Once identified, that name is seen as the "life program" of that person. For example, *Malidoma* means "he who makes friends with the stranger." Somé's name fore-shadowed that he would spend his life living, working, and teaching in other cultures.

Donna was unable to discover where I had hidden the lit-tle doll that symbolized her soul until she called out "Juanita," the name she had been given at birth. My ances-tors who lived in Mexico would not name a child until it was born. Even then, the parents did not choose the name. The curandera, who was able to look deeply into the child and ob-serve his or her soul, would choose the correct one. My teacher Ehekateotl has taught me that the Aztecs still name their children by using the Aztec calendar. For example, I was born on the year that begins with the "flower day," the day called Xochitl. When I joined the tribe, I was given this name in a beautiful ceremony. Alicia Gaspar de Alba speaks eloquently about the importance of names in her book *Women's Voices from the Borderlands:* "Only by seeding the new world with the old names will the memories come back."

When I do a soul retrieval, I always call out my client's name, using many different pitches and tones of voice. I never call in an angry voice because as children our parents may have scared our little souls by yelling out our names in anger. If clients feel that their name is "tainted" and/or not a true reflection of who they are, I help them choose a new name or a spirit name. For example, I do not go by my first name, Ada, because it was my mother's name and still carries too much negative energy for me.

My own name has gone through several permutations during my lifetime. First I anglicized it to Helen, the name given to me in the hospital by the doctors and nurses who helped me to recover from hepatitis. When I went to make a new life for myself in Los Angeles, I returned to Elena, which symbolically allowed me to retrieve a part of my Chicana soul. When I reached the age of fifty-two, the end of my first cycle of life, my Aztec tribe gave me the name Xochitlwetzkapahtli, which means "flower that brings medicine through laughter." This name embodies my essence as a healer and a woman, and the beauty of the tradition that I have reclaimed. It is a name that I am proud to bear.

Soul Retrievals Are as Diverse as the Soul

Not all soul retrievals are as dramatic as Donna's, nor do I always know what part of the soul needs to be retrieved. Not all parts of the soul want to come out of hiding. Some souls tell me, when I see them during a trance journey, that they are truly fine where they are. I always make it a habit to tell my clients that whatever happens, happens. If we find nothing, or don't find what we expect to find, that's okay too. There are no hard and fast rules about this process. I remember one experience with Gloria, a young Chicana in her early twenties who came to see me because she had suffered sexual abuse as a child and wanted a soul retrieval. As we worked together, we were able to pinpoint that she had been sexually molested at age three. Fortunately she'd had a pretty good upbringing and was healthy, so we didn't have a lot of issues to work through. She had seen me lecture at a nearby nursing school, and she was ready to do the necessary work.

I went on a trance journey with the preconceived notion that I was going to find the molested three-year-old. Instead, to my surprise, I found myself in a river. I went deep under the water and discovered a *viejita,* an old grandmother, holding a small child of five years old in her arms. The child was very pale and very still. In Spanish, the *viejita* said, "Here, you are a nurse, give her CPR. She's drowning." I took the child from her arms, brought her up to the surface of the water, laid her on the bank, and resuscitated her. I didn't see the *viejita* anymore, so I just held the child until she was breathing normally.

When I returned from my journey and told Gloria the story, she looked at me wide-eyed as if she couldn't believe it. She said, "Oh, my God, I had completely forgotten that I almost drowned as a child." She told me that, when she was about five or six years old, she and her family had been picnicking along the banks of the Rio Grande. Her father had warned her not to play alongside the river but, being a little kid, she had disobeyed him and fallen in. She couldn't even remember who had pulled her out.

She was very close to her grandmother, who had died two or three years after the near drowning, and it had great meaning for her that I had seen her during my trance journey. She said, "My *abuelita* was taking care of that part of my soul until you came for it." To me, this made perfect sense. I said, "Of course we needed to get the five-year-old soul that stayed in that river before we could get to the three-year-old who was molested."

So you never know in what order the things are going to happen. Maybe we need to go and retrieve the part of the soul that we left behind six months ago, or the part that suffered *justo* at age two. It all depends on what our soul needs at the time. Since the soul is sacred, and my job is not to control other people's actions or prejudge their needs, I try to be as receptive as possible when I take people through their soul's journey.

Catherine: "I Don't Want to Be a Hearth Goddess"

Catherine didn't have as dramatic a soul retrieval as Donna, but the work we did together was exactly what her soul needed. Catherine is one of the most beautiful human beings I have ever seen. Almost angelic in appearance, she has peach-colored skin, blond hair, and blue eyes. The first time we met she told me that one of her role models was Aphrodite, the love goddess, whom she admired because of her ability to be both a mother and a free woman. In the Greek myth, Aphrodite's children would be angry with her when she was gone for long periods of time, but would always be happy to see her when she came home, forgetting that she had ever left. "I'd rather be like Aphrodite than a hearth goddess," she told me. "I envy traditional wives, but I also want to be alone when I need to be. What I have to offer my mate is excitement and adventure."

Despite what she said, Catherine's soul liked to swing between the two extremes of homebody and glamorous risk taker. Sometimes she would come in and tell me that she was really getting into baking cookies, wanting to get pregnant, keeping house, and doing all the things that hearth goddesses in the Greek myths loved to do. Other times, she would say, "Well, I went out and had a few drinks with this guy I've known for a while, and I'm thinking of having an affair with him." Even the way she dressed swung from one side of the pendulum to the other. Sometimes she would come to see me looking very sexy with pink streaks in her hair and long lacy skirts. Other times she would wear flowing granny dresses and bring me some of her homemade brownies.

My job was to figure out which person Catherine really was, in terms of her soul. During our first soul retrieval, all we found was a withdrawn, sad child who didn't want to talk and certainly didn't want to return to Catherine. One of the very important things that Catherine said to me at the time was, "I don't want to end up like my mom." For the purpose of uncovering Catherine's real soul, we had to work through all of her dysfunctions that were very much like her mother's.

Catherine grew up in New Zealand. Her half-Maori mother, Erica, was a diagnosed manic-depressive and was often hospitalized for this condition. Erica was once hospitalized for two years. She also had an eating disorder that caused her to swing between extremes of thinness and fatness, she was a compulsive shopper, and often experienced bouts of *bilis*, rage. Although Catherine was fair in her coloring, her mother had short, dark wavy hair and looked like a Native American. Even though the pressure to assimilate to white culture was great, Erica kept many Maori customs and even went to the Maori church.

Erica's parents had had high expectations for their daughter. They wouldn't let her play with the other children, and made her practice the piano for long hours. When she failed her college exams at age sixteen, Erica felt a great deal of shame, as if she had let her parents down, failing to live up to their ambitions for her.

Catherine's mom and her alcoholic father would sometimes physically abuse her, and her mother seemed emotionally absent much of the time. "Mom would withdraw often," she told me. "I remember her being there, but not there. I always felt so empty when I was with her. She would pick me up at school and we would walk the five miles home without saying anything. I would be afraid to talk to her, to make her angry." Sometimes, her mother would yell at her and hit her, saying things like, "You think you're pretty, don't you? Well, you're ugly. No man will ever love you."

Catherine was very emotionally enmeshed with her mother, and put a lot of energy into trying to avoid being like her in any way. Once, when she had seen a picture of her mother as a little girl, she noticed that she had very sad eyes. She told me, "I know my grandmother never shared affection with my mother. She only kissed my mother twice in her whole life. But my grandmother is Maori, the culture is rooted in the earth. I think my grandmother wanted my mother to be successful in a white man's world. Maybe they stopped honoring their culture. My great-grandmother discouraged her kids from speaking Maori at home. Even today my great-aunt pretends that she doesn't understand Maori, when she understands it perfectly."

When Catherine was twenty-one, her mother died of a drug overdose. Catherine went through the Maori funeral custom of having the body in the house for three days, and told me that this helped her to grieve.

The months that followed brought about many changes in rapid succession. Shortly after her mother's death, Catherine moved to New Mexico, and five months later she was raped. Three months after the rape, she met her husband in a bar, and six weeks later she moved in with him.

From the start, her relationship with her husband was erratic, and she had very ambivalent feelings about him. One part of her wanted to stay in the marriage forever, and another part wanted to explore other things. Catherine had no clear plans about her future. She would tell me that she wanted to finish college, and then she'd go and enroll in a creative writing course and work hard. But she would also go through periods when she would drink too much and eat compulsively. She frequently vacillated between wanting to have children and wanting to leave her marriage.

Catherine's Soul Retrievals

Catherine and I identified many *justos* in her life, many insults to her soul. She had become bulimic when she was fourteen years old, and started drinking alcohol in her teens. She resented the fact that her father had never stood up to her abusive mother or protected Catherine when her mother hurt her. There were times when she felt so bad that she had run away from home. When she was eleven, she was sexually abused by a relative while her mother was in the hospital. Around this time she became terrified of the dark because she had frequent nightmares. Every night she would pray to Jesus, pleading, "Please, Jesus, don't let me have a bad dream," but Jesus never answered her prayers. Catherine told me she thought she had bad dreams because she was a bad girl. This was important information, because it showed me one of the reasons why Catherine did not have a balanced relationship with parts of her soul. Why would you want to have a relationship with yourself if you thought you were bad?

During Catherine's first soul retrieval, she saw a lion who said he was one of her guides. She also saw an old crone, a mischievous fairy, and Aphrodite's face. These beings took her to a grave that she felt was her husband's. Facing toward the east, she placed flowers on it. Then she saw herself packing up her house and moving to another state where she was looking for a place to stay and a job.

After this soul retrieval, we talked about some of the things she had experienced during her trance journey. I told her that it seemed as if she was saying good-bye to her marriage; and that her soul, even though it was scared, really wanted to leave her husband and explore what it was like to be single. Catherine was in a child-parent role with her husband. She was the child. Part of the reason for this was that she had married him too soon after her mother's suicide and her own rape. She had needed protection back then because she was feeling lost and vulnerable, but now she was growing up and was better able to take care of herself. She told me, "I felt sad when I went through my journey, but I knew that my feelings weren't coming from a place of depression, they were coming from my higher power."

Although there was nothing earthshaking about this soul retrieval, it seemed very useful and practical, and I knew that Catherine's mind and feelings had been very present during it. In soul retrievals, it's important to remember that you will not always have a dramatic experience. In Catherine's case, I would have expected her to see a little lost, abused child, but there were other parts of her that needed to be addressed first before she could get to the younger, injured parts of her soul. This is just another example of the uniqueness of each person's soul, the individual ways of experiencing this process.

Three months later, we did find the lost child within Catherine. She and I saw a very small child huddled in the dark, naked, frightened, and freezing. She was emaciated and I could see all the bones sticking out of her back. Even though she was starving, she was too scared to ask for anything. This little girl thought she was invisible, and that no one could see her. She was crying soundlessly.

One of the things that Catherine said about this particular soul retrieval was, "Elena, I don't know how to love that part of my soul. I feel so clumsy. I push her back into the darkness where my parents pushed me. I tell myself that I'm not good enough, not slim enough, not pretty enough, and I seek outside validation to affirm myself. It's taken me one whole year to hear what you are trying to tell me. I have to learn how to be a mother to my own little injured soul. When I eat compulsively, I am force-feeding that part of me. When I diet, I starve her."

A few months later, we had another soul retrieval. In this one she saw her Auntie Mae, her grandmother's sister on her mother's side. To Catherine, this woman was like a grandmother. The old woman hugged and kissed her, and said, "Oh, Catherine, you look so lovely." When Catherine first saw her she felt sad, and told her, "Grandmother, you were never grumpy. You were always there taking care of us, cooking us good meals when Mum was in the hospital. I want to learn about my Maori roots, I miss them." In her trance, she started to dance around her grandmother, feeling like a woman warrior.

Afterward, during the *plática*, Catherine told me that this journey had shown her that she had been loved. Even though her own parents had not been there for her in the way she would have liked, she had received consistent love from her Auntie Mae. To me, this meant that she had enough love in her soul to love herself. If we know that we are loved, then we can also love. As Catherine's ancestors were beginning to speak to her, she was also starting to realize that her Maori culture had the medicine to help her to heal herself. Auntie Mae had died when she was almost ninety years old, and she said that she wished that she had learned about her Maori roots from her. Catherine was truly starting to bring back parts of her lost soul.

In her final soul retrieval, we found a two-and-a-half-year-old girl wandering around on the moon. She was very neglected, dirty, and autistic. Her spirit guide was a dragon with wings, and he brought her back down to earth. After this soul retrieval, Catherine felt nauseated and vomited, which to me is always a sign that someone has returned into her body. This kind of vomiting is a way to bring the soul back to earth, to ground, to bring that lost part back into the body. It was a true spiritual cleansing.

Shortly after this soul retrieval, Catherine went back to New Zealand for a few months. When she visited her mother's grave, she was able to realize that her mother *did* love her but, most important she realized that she was separate from her mother. She also discovered that she was ready to become a mother herself, integrating the hearth goddess and Aphrodite into her one soul. She conceived shortly after that, and her son was born in New Zealand. A few months later the lost little girl grew up and divorced her husband. Because I knew that Catherine needed a strong community of women, I invited her to a gathering of medicine women of several spiritual belief systems. One of the participants was a Hawaiian medicine woman who, because the Maori and the Hawaiians come from the same genetic stock, acknowledged Catherine as a relative. This experience was very empowering to Catherine. She also met a Wiccan priestess to whom she decided to apprentice herself. Since then, Catherine has become a Wiccan priestess herself and is teaching Celtic history at a university. She is happily remarried to a man from New Zealand, and is raising two young sons. She loves being a hearth goddess and she loves being Aphrodite, the love goddess.

Family Soul Retrievals

Another type of soul retrieval that I do is a family soul retrieval. One woman came to see me after her teenaged son had been fatally knifed. She had already lost a three-year-old child and the shock of losing a second child froze a part of her soul so that she was unable to mourn him. Many Chicano mothers will release their grief in an earthy, grounded, complete manner by trying to throw themselves onto the coffin or into the grave. In this way, they are able to express the despair of their loss fully and begin to empty their hearts of anguish so that they can truly begin to heal. This woman felt numb at her son's funeral. She just couldn't find that part of herself that needed to mourn. As time went on, she began to feel more and more listless and hopeless. Her family became concerned when she began to get very sick with fainting spells and seizurelike activity. Before she came to me, she had been given CAT scans, brain scans, and blood tests, but no one was able to find anything organically wrong with her. One of her doctors suggested that she take antidepressant medication, but she refused.

Eight months after her son's death, this woman came to see me as a last resort. During the *plática*, I realized that she was not coming to see me to help her to grieve, but to see if I could help her with her physical problems. This is one of the reasons that the *plática* is such a good tool. It often helps me to uncover the *real* root of the problem, not what the person *thinks* is the problem.

It was clear to me that what this woman really needed to do was to grieve the loss of her son. Since she was unable to do so, a part of her soul had stayed in the coffin with him. Her husband and daughter were present at this meeting, and one of the things that I discovered was that her husband was very protective of her. Without meaning to, he was keeping her from grieving. Every time she would light a candle for her son, he would tell her, "Just let him go on. Lighting candles is keeping him from evolving spiritually." The few times she was able to cry, he'd tell her to be strong and not to cry.

If possible, it is always better to go to the place where the *susto* occurred. I felt that it was important that we do a soul retrieval at her son's grave site, and the family agreed to go along with this. First I did a ceremony for the mother, burning copal and flicking my eagle feather over her entire body. She started to have intense pain in her womb, and doubled over with it. Her husband immediately tried to rush to her side to help her up, but I stopped him. By this time she was kneeling over her son's grave. The body is very wise and knows exactly what it needs to do. Her fainting spells had been telling her that she needed to go back into that earthy place where she had left her soul.

I asked her, "When your son's casket was being lowered into the ground, what did your soul really want to do?"

She let out a wail that came from the depths of her soul, and threw herself down prostrate on the ground. She started to scream, over and over, "*Mijito, mijito,* please don't leave me." There it was. That's where she had left her soul, in the grave with her son. She couldn't bring him back into her womb and give him life again, so her soul had wanted to die with him. I told her gently that it was not her time, that she had other children, a husband, and grandchildren whom she loved very dearly, and who needed her very much. Her husband learned from this experience that it was very important for his wife to cry. From then on when she lit candles and wept for her son, he told her, "Light as many candles as you want. Only a mother knows what her son needs."

Group Soul Retrieval

For five years I have given a workshop at Ghost Ranch and other locations for health-care professionals who wanted to learn about curanderismo in a more hands-on, experiential sort of way. I usually get about thirty participants, often from all over the United States. Called The Dance of the Curanderos, this workshop introduces participants to the techniques used in *limpias, pláticas,* and soul retrievals. I especially stress how important it is for healers to pay attention to the areas in their own lives that need healing. Soul retrievals are an important part of this process because it is difficult to heal others if you are missing parts of yourself. While it is unrealistic to ask healers to be perfect, since all of us carry *sustos* in our hearts, we need to work on ourselves consistently. To be of service to others, we need to have a strong sense of self. For that reason, I always have those who attend the workshop participate in a group soul retrieval.

Group soul retrievals can be very powerful because they help us realize the universality of our wounds and traumas. In groups of this size, the *plática* takes the form of a talking circle in which I pass an eagle feather to each participant and ask them to share their wounds and where they feel that they have lost a part of their souls.

In one soul retrieval, I had asked all participants to bring a doll with them that symbolized the lost part of their soul. I instructed them to carry that doll with them throughout the whole weekend experience—to sleep with it and take it into the cafeteria for meals.

On a Sunday afternoon, we did a soul retrieval. With their heads toward the center of the circle, each person lay down and made him- or herself comfortable. My assistants and I were in the inner circle and the participants surrounded us like the spokes of a wheel. My helpers played various percussion and musical instruments, such as drums and rain sticks, and the workshop participants held their doll to their hearts as I guided them into a shamanic journey. I led them to their animal and human guides, and asked these spiritual beings to find the lost soul part and to bring it back to the man or woman. After all of the participants returned from their jour-

ney, I asked them to give me their dolls. As I sat there surrounded by all of them, I felt like one of those clay Pueblo fig-
urines of a mama sitting with babies all around her.

One at a time, I held up a doll, and said, "Who is this?"
Each person would say his name, and then tell the group
about the part of his soul that the doll represented. For example, someone might say, "Pablito is very shy and has felt
ashamed since he was a little boy because he is so dark
skinned. The kids at school used to make fun of him, calling
him '*negrito.*' When I went on my journey, I found him all
alone in a corner, huddled up in a fetal position, sobbing. I
went to him, held him in my arms, and comforted him, telling
him that I'm not going to let anybody hurt him anymore. I
told him that it was okay that he was so dark skinned, and
that he is beautiful just the way he is."

There are certain things human beings have to learn as a
gut-level body experience. We can't learn everything with
our intellects. Even though it had been embarrassing for
these thirty well-educated health-care practitioners to carry a
doll around with them all day, in front of all the other people
who were attending workshops at Ghost Ranch that weekend, by the end of their soul retrievals, they were hugging
that doll as if it were a *real* part of themselves. This experience
always reminds me of the story *The Velveteen Rabbit.* When the
rabbit asked the wise Skin Horse, "Does it hurt to be real?"
the Skin Horse answered, "Sometimes," for he always told
the truth. But he also added, "When you are real, you don't
mind being hurt." It is always infinitely better for human beings to suffer the pain of finding out who they really are because the rewards and freedoms always outweigh the pain
they have to undergo to get there.

Can We Do Our Own Soul Retrievals?

Many people ask me if it is possible for us to do our own soul retrievals. While we can't do very deep soul retrievals for ourselves, because we need a deep sense of community to support us on those kinds of journeys, we can do some soul retrieval work alone if we have a good sense of self.

A friend of mine had recently broken up with her boyfriend after a two-year long-distance relationship in which they each took turns staying in the other's home. When my friend spent time at her boyfriend's house in California, one of their favorite places was his kitchen. He loved the blue corn atole cereal that she would make for him every morning. They would sit in their chairs in his small cozy kitchen, having breakfast and spending many wonderful hours talking and laughing. She especially loved his old-fashioned stove with a metal railing around the outside of it.

A few months after the breakup, and despite many letting-go ceremonies, my friend continued to feel an emptiness that told her she had left a part of her soul in her ex-lover's home. Knowing intuitively that she had to go back there and retrieve it, she lit her candles, smudged herself with copal, lay down in a safe place, and went into a trance. She entered his house through the front door, and went through his living room and dining room. When she reached the kitchen, she saw herself standing there in front of the stove making blue corn atole. When she told that part of her soul that she had come for it, it grabbed the railing of the stove in a death grip and said, "I don't want to go with you." My friend told her soul that she needed it, and that if she had to take her soul out of there forcibly, she would. She literally went up behind the lost part of her soul and put her arms around it, lifting it up and carrying it out of the kitchen. She told her soul, "I will take care of you. The relationship is over and he can no longer fulfill that part of you. I know that this is very sad, but I will comfort your sadness." That afternoon, her ex-lover called her and said, "You were here, weren't you?" Crying softly, he said, "I know that you came back for that part of your soul that you had left here, because the house feels very empty without you." That confirmation was one of his parting gifts to her.

The soul doesn't always leave the body because we have had a traumatic or sad experience. Sometimes a part of us wants to stay behind in a place where we have been very happy. Every time I leave Ghost Ranch after a weekend workshop, I have to do a soul retrieval for myself because a part of my soul is reluctant to leave such a beautiful place. Situated in the high desert mountains of northern New Mexico, Ghost Ranch is one of the most spiritual places that I have ever been. Georgia O'Keeffe lived and died there, and the surrounding desert and hills inspired her to create many of her incredible paintings. It is a sacred power place for me.

I remember a particular Sunday afternoon when I was driving home after spending the weekend working with a group of remarkable people. The farther away from Ghost Ranch I got, the more I began to feel an emptiness inside that told me that something was missing. Several of my friends from out of state had participated in the workshop and were spending the night with me before heading home in the morning. When we got back to my place, I asked them to help me do a soul retrieval and bring back that part of myself that had stayed behind.

They all gathered around my bed and started calling out, "Elena, Elenita, come back. Come back." I had my eyes closed, and I saw that part of me flying and whirling in the incredible skies above Ghost Ranch, hopping from star to star and feeling so much at home there. I silently told that part of me, "I know you love it there, but I need you here with me. We will go back there many times, but right now, I need you." At that moment, my compadre Guillermo put his hand on my chest and my third eye, and I felt Elena return. I started to sob and all my compadres and comadres put their hands on a part of my body and soothed me as if I were a small child. They all said, "Welcome home, Elenita, welcome home." They covered me up with blankets, tucked me in, kissed me good night, and turned out the light. I fell sound asleep.

After the many hundreds of soul retrievals that I've done, it amazes me that Western medicine still has not realized the importance of the soul and spirit in healing. My clients have been such powerful teachers to me about how illnesses of the body, mind, and heart are so deeply interconnected with the many soul losses we have experienced. They have shown me how a strong spirit and soul can allow us the resiliency to bounce back from great physical and emotional trauma. I do believe, however, that the modern medical profession is slowly waking up to these ideas. More and more medical schools are incorporating mind-and-body healing into their curriculums, and nursing schools are teaching transcultural and holistic nursing. But we still have a long way to go. My vision is that one day the curandera in the white lab coat will unite with the curandera with the eagle feather.

Chapter Five

The Twisted Heart

Where is your heart
If you give your heart to each and every thing,
you lead it nowhere . . . you destroy your heart.
— *Nezahualcóyotl, Aztec poet*

In Nahuatl the word *heart* is derived from the same root as the word *movement*, and this poem tells us that seeking and desiring those earthly things that are not of real value will result in loss of the energetic, potent, and true self. When we are envious of an aspect of another person, be it her job, her physical appearance, or her accomplishments, a big chunk of our energy goes toward wishing for what we do not have.

Women often feel envy around weight issues. A slightly

overweight, attractive Chicana in her early thirties came to me for help complaining of weight gain, depression, and numbness of feeling. She told me that she had become depressed shortly after her best friend lost twenty pounds. At that point, she began to find fault with everything her friend did. She was starting to hate her friend, and she began hating herself for feeling this way. These feelings were tying up her emotions in a way that was making it hard for her to go to work and take care of her family. The vicious cycle of envy was also contributing to her gaining weight because she overate when she felt depressed.

Another client, the grandmother of a friend, told me that she had lit a perpetual candle in the hopes of decreasing the envy of her neighbors. She worked as a maid and her grateful employers always gave her their unwanted clothes. Because she was always so well dressed, her neighbors had begun calling her Manuela *la farsante* (Manuela the snob), even though she was just as poor as her neighbors. Manuela was investing a lot of her emotional energy in worrying about losing the friendship and good opinion of her neighbors.

We need 100 percent of our energy to live our lives in a healthy way, just as we need 100 percent of our souls. When we are suffering from envy, what we are really experiencing is a type of soul loss. People with envy were once innocent and trusting, but the traumas of life have diverted their path into a passive role of wishing, giving them the false expectation that someday their frog will turn into a prince. Soul loss comes from childhood deprivation, hunger, and wounding.

We Are All Born with Legitimate Needs

Envy can stem from normal impulses. We are all born with needs that are legitimate and should be satisfied as we grow into maturity, but many of us have instead been raised in families where no one has received adequate love, understanding, or encouragement for *generations.* This causes us to leave the nest hungry.

A forty-year-old Native American named Polito came to me suffering from a terrible envy of those whose family lives reflected warmth and closeness. Polito had lived a life of neglect and isolation. His father had died when he was seven years old, and his little sister had died seven months after. When he was eight years old, he was sent to an Indian boarding school because his alcoholic mother was unable to take care of him. She was often abusive, and he could never remember her smiling or touching him in a loving way. He told me shortly after I met him, "I never felt wanted by anyone. Nobody went to my high school graduation, and when I left for Vietnam, no one came to see me off."

Polito sought closeness in the wrong places. He had been in relationships with two women who had been very abusive to him, just as his mother had been. These women were never able to make a commitment to him, but just kept him dangling. He had never married or had children, even though he envied married men and fathers. As an alcoholic who had been in trouble with the law for drunk driving, he envied people who could relax with a few drinks socially without going overboard. During the week of the Superbowl, he told me that he was envious of people who could sit down and watch the game, sharing a few beers with their friends. He felt cut off from friendship.

Ironically, the depression, sadness, and envy he felt had finally built up to the point where he began drinking again after five years of sobriety. This was one of the reasons he came to me. He was caught drinking while driving and had lost his license. He was so out of control that he came drunk to his first therapy session.

Polito wasted a lot of time wishing for the things that he did not have, the ability to have friends and enjoy social drinking with them, the need to have a family and children. When his envy became too painful for him to bear, he fed it with alcoholism, abusive relationships, and self-destructive behaviors. His envy imploded. Like Polito, we often punish ourselves when we feel envy.

Envy Has Consequences

Since we all have "energy bodies" as well as physical bodies, we are all continually sending out negative and positive thought and energy to other persons and things around us, often in a mindless way. We often do not think of the consequences that these thoughts and vibrations have on all living things. My teacher Ehekateotl has explained that we can pray for good things to happen to others, or we can pray for bad things. When we pray, this is one way of focusing our energy into an intent. For instance, we might be watching a friend dancing the salsa really well and getting a lot of attention. One part of us is admiring her, but another part of us is envious, silently praying, "I hope she trips and makes a fool out of herself." These kinds of thoughts are so unconscious, we might not even notice them at the time. We may be completely unaware that our thoughts could be hurting someone, but they are. Christ taught that negative *thoughts* were just as bad as negative *actions*. Whether we agree with such a pure interpretation or not, when we make others the intense focus of our lust, malice, resentment, and longings, our energy does have the potential to harm them.

Envy can make us physically, emotionally, and spiritually sick. It has the potential of making our object of desire ill as well. For these reasons, envy has an impact on the object of desire, the envied. The envious person creates an intrusive bond with the person she envies, and that bond can be destructive to both. Some individuals are totally unaware that they are sending out envious thoughts to other people because they do not recognize that the feelings they are projecting are envious.

For example, a student might hide her envious feelings toward her teacher by bringing him special gifts and making herself indispensable. But underneath, her envy will make her highly sensitive to anything the teacher says about her, perceiving it all as criticism. No matter what the teacher says or does, she will find fault with her and tell the other students that the teacher does not appreciate her.

Envy is an *interaction* between two people, the one who envies and the one who is the object of envy. People we envy are a constant reminder of what is missing in our lives, and sometimes we wish them harm, or even worse, we want to get rid of them. A person whose heart is twisted with envy has the potential of being a soul thief. When ice skater Tonya Harding hired thugs to break Nancy Kerrigan's legs, she was injuring Kerrigan where it hurt the most—in her soul. Because of this injury, Kerrigan almost lost her chance of competing in the Olympics. And Harding certainly destroyed an important part of her own life when she was convicted of harming her rival and disqualified from competing. I believe that Selena, the young Tejana singer from Corpus Christi, Texas, was murdered due to *envídia*. The woman who killed her started out as her fan and then became her manager. She envied Selena because she herself had always wanted to be a singer, and also because Selena was so much more attractive than she was. "Near a star, be a star" is the sick chant of envious fans.

Envy is a natural emotion. All of us have felt the twinges of envy at someone else's good fortune. I like to say jokingly that 99 percent of the population has envy and the other 1 percent is lying. We generally do not like to admit that we feel envious of others.

Degrees of Envy

The feelings generated by *envídia* are both broad and specific to the individual personality. Since envy is a normal feeling, this condition can range from mild to severe. *Envídia* actually produces physical sensations that we might be aware of, a tight feeling in the heart area, a twist in the place between breaths. Envy often catches us completely off guard. When we hear that a friend has won the lottery, we notice that our smile is frozen when we congratulate her, and we're not sure why. We feel an uncomfortable twinge in the chest area, an uneasiness that we want to ignore or repress because we unconsciously feel shame around envy because it is such a naked emotion. We know that we love our friend, but something is happening to us, flooding us with feelings that make us uncomfortable. We feel sad, and we don't know why. There is a tremendous denial in envy because we do not want to acknowledge that we can be greedy, spiteful, judging, critical, vengeful, selfish, manipulative, resentful, and all of the horrible traits we only see in others.

A good climate for *envídia* to develop is when the gap between the rich and the poor widens. Envy grows in people who must spend decades living from hand to mouth. When I was a child, I always got my sister Irma's hand-me-downs, including her old shoes. I hated wearing shoes that pinched my toes and dresses that were not my style. I would feel envious every time Irma got a new dress or a new pair of shoes. I still have remnants of these feelings, which result in my having a closet full of clothes and shoes of all styles and colors. This kind of situation is very common. People often wonder, "Why am I spending money on all of this stuff?" or "Why do I have all of this food in my refrigerator when I end up having to throw half of it away?" Some people go into debt by overcharging on their credit cards, eating at expensive restaurants, or spending money on things that they think they need to have in order to compete with their neighbors, but they don't know why. They don't realize that this hunger they have inside comes from a time when their souls were deprived. They are going after the wrong kinds of "food" to fill up the empty places inside, when what they really want is to regain the lost parts of their souls.

In Mexico, envy is one of the most commonly recognized

diseases. In the *mercados*, one can buy a variety of oils, po-
tions, amulets, soaps, or herbs to prevent or offset the effects
of envy. If a person falls victim to *envídia*, curanderos perform
a variety of rituals to cure the patient. This is not to say that
Mexico suffers more envy than any other country, but that
this disease has been assimilated into the cultural beliefs as a
disharmony that affects mind, body, and spirit. In Mexican
culture, there are many variations on the story in which a
person sells his soul to the devil to get something that he envies. When the devil comes to collect, however, the person
tricks him out of his prize because he has learned his lesson
and realized the true value of his soul.

Metaphorically I see envy as a kind of highly contagious,
dangerous virus. This can be seen in the way that the disharmony caused by envy seems to spread. The particular type of
envy spawned by the overwhelming materialism of the U.S.
has begun to trickle down into Latin America, permeating the
borders between cultures. The spread of this virus can be
seen in the fact that so many young people in Mexico today,
who used to be content with themselves the way they are, are
now starting to envy the people in the U.S. They are watching the material opulence imported by American television
programs, listening to the values expressed in American music, copying our expensive clothes and athletic shoes, wishing
for cell phones, computers, and other electronic equipment.
What must they do to get all of this stuff and how are they going to pay for it? Are they going to sell their souls for it, losing the very cultural values that have kept them healthy and
in balance? Today there is a real fear that Mexican teenagers
will literally sell their souls to the devil by starting to deal
drugs and/or commit petty crimes to get the things they think

they need. They are already doing so in ever-increasing numbers. In the U.S. a huge crime rate among adolescents is already a reality. Teenagers from economically disadvantaged neighborhoods say, "Why should we work at McDonald's for minimum wage when we can sell drugs and make hundreds of dollars a day?"

In the U.S. we are discovering that few of the things that the media promises will make us happy really do have that power. The envy generated by the hunger for material possessions has reached epic proportions. Parents are tired of buying their kids $150 athletic shoes, expensive computers so they can play all the computer games and get on the Internet, and even fancy cars. In Dallas the favorite graduation present for affluent high school girls is a nose job or a breast implant. These things are done so that these young women can be as attractive as other girls whom they envy.

The Six Roots of Envy

In my many years of practice as a curandera, I have noticed that there are six main things that people envy: power, money, beauty, body shape, love, and youth. Men seem to envy power and money more, whereas women become obsessed with the other qualities.

Men tend to feel envy of other men's appearance, especially in the areas of hair and height. I once treated a man who spent a great deal of time obsessing about his toupee. He was also upset because he stood only five feet four inches tall. When it was windy, he always wore a baseball cap. Swimming was out of the question because he feared that people would notice that he was wearing a hairpiece. He spent hours looking in the mirror and trying to fix his hair so that it would look natural.

This man was horribly envious of men who were tall and had a full head of hair. He had lost his hair in his early twenties, and now he was in his forties. Whenever he began to date a new woman, he would worry about whether or not she would find out that he was wearing a toupee. I told him that she probably knew this the first time that they went out together, and that she had already made the decision to continue dating him because she liked him.

When I suggested to this man that he just take off his toupee and accept the fact that he was bald, he became very shamefaced and confessed to me that he couldn't do that. He had received a botched hair transplant and had so many terrible scars on his head that he felt like he was forever stuck with the toupee. Unfortunately, I was unable to help him. The man felt so vulnerable after showing me his scars that he never returned to see me. This demonstrated to me how desperately his energy was tied up with his worries about being bald. He had never had a stable relationship with a woman because his obsession with his hair filled him with a terror of being emotionally and physically close. I couldn't help thinking, "What a sad waste of twenty years."

Women spend a tremendous amount of time and money on weight-loss programs, exercise, plastic surgery, and cosmetics to make them look younger. I have found that the more a woman obsesses about her body, the less she lives in it. Women who are anorexic or overweight and constantly dieting are not fully present in their bodies. We are all born with certain physical traits that we inherit. Once we start rejecting the shape that we were born with, we begin to lose that intuitive part of our nature. Many times it is unrealistic to want to become a size 8, or whatever our goal may be. Our bodies naturally tell us what to eat, and when, in order to remain healthy. When we are hungry, we are supposed to have a meal; when we are full, we are supposed to stop eating. When we tamper with that natural appestat of our souls, the system breaks down. There is an incredible wholeness and satisfaction about accepting your body just the way it is. Clarissa Pinkola Estes, who is a large woman, praises the woman who feels the richness of her body celebrating the earth. When I met Estes in person, her energy was so grounded and vibrant that I knew I was looking at a woman who was joyously at home in her body.

Envy of the Perfect Relationship

The vast number of people who come to me are either dissatisfied with their current relationship or still under the illusion that the perfect man or woman is going to arrive someday and save them. When they watch young couples holding hands or see romantic movies, they feel as if their relationships, past and present, just don't measure up. Some of them even ask me if I can give them a love potion or read tarot cards to help them find their soul mate. Somehow they believe that if they can only perform the right magical action, they will meet the person they are looking for.

A relationship is part of your life, but it should not be your whole life. When people are obsessed with finding the perfect relationship that will feed all of their hungers or satisfy all of their needs, they forget to look within their own souls for nourishment. These people will go to their graves very hungry.

I once worked with a client named David, a handsome, single Italian-American man around the age of thirty-four. David asked me if I had a love potion to offer him because he was tired of being alone. Several months before he came to see me, he had started to withdraw from other people and spend more time alone in his apartment. He had become more and more melancholy, and his energy had gotten very low. "I feel anxious," he told me, "because I want to meet my soul mate, have kids, and be happy."

As time went on, David became obsessed with the couples he saw on the street, at the malls, and at his job as a construction worker. He stared at beautiful couples, noticing their body language, and felt his heart wrench when he saw them looking at each other, kissing, or holding hands. If he was at the shopping mall, he would invariably notice all the couples. He would single one out and follow the pair around for a while because, in a strange way, he wanted to feel as if he were part of the loving energy that they generated. Those coveted relationships became food for his fantasies, which were all romantic vignettes of him and his future "beloved." He was torn between wanting to stay home and be alone with his fantasies, and obsessing about how he was ever going to meet the love of his life if he did not go out. He was constantly ruminating about his dilemma, which, in turn, made him more uncertain about what to do.

After we had done a series of *limpias*, David clearly saw

that he had allowed himself to become involved in a vicious cycle. He began to ask himself honest and grounded questions, such as, "Do I really want to be in a relationship? Am I ready for one?" Once he had made this commitment to explore what was in his heart, we took his confusion to Spirit. He began to pray quite honestly for clarity and realized that he was ambivalent about getting that close to someone. The responsibilities of being a father appeared overwhelming to him at this time in his life, and he feared losing those special times he spent alone, which were vital to him. On the other hand, he saw how lonely he was. He knew that his biological clock was ticking , telling him, "I want a baby!" People do not think that men have biological clocks, but they do. I have seen many male patients who express a strong desire to have children and begin to feel desperate when they have reached their thirties and still have not found a mate. Some of these men perceive babies as a means to carry on their names, others long to have children before they get "old."

One thing he was sure of, the time that he was spending on fantasy was a waste of his energy. David truly wanted to love deeply and be loved deeply in return. He wanted a family of his own, but he was fearful of losing his blessed solitude. After a few more *pláticas* and *limpias*, he began to integrate all of the contradictory yearnings in his soul and heart, and his path became clear to him. The envious feelings he had experienced toward loving couples had uncovered an important message: "You are not happy. Do something. You really *do* want a relationship. You are just scared."

After realizing what he really wanted and needed, David made a commitment to stop obsessing about other couples, stop fantasizing, and stop isolating himself from others. He knew that his heart truly desired a family, but he also realized that he was fearful of the unknown. Acknowledging this made it possible for him to work through his fears. Only at that point was David genuinely ready to start looking for a relationship.

Envy Is a Mirror

Envy can serve a positive purpose as well as a negative one. When you are within the "normal" range of envy, the things you desire act as mirrors, messengers from your heart telling you what your soul most desires. Although envy can be incredibly destructive, it can also tell us what makes us happy, healthy, and loving. At such times, it is our job to listen.

If you envy a public speaker, perhaps there is a part of your soul that yearns to teach, to speak to a group about what you know. You know that you have something to say that is bottled up inside of you. If you envy a co-worker who was recently promoted, perhaps you are feeling stuck in your current position and feel ready for new challenges in your job. If you covet another person's wealth and material possessions, perhaps your life is not rich enough emotionally and spiritually.

Pure undiluted feelings like envy become little signposts to the intuitive aspects of our personality. They send a message to the mind, giving us the opportunity to analyze the emotions we are experiencing. They offer us great opportunities for growth and change, if we are willing to listen. When we are out of balance and our hearts are twisted with envy, our intuition is not accessible to us. When we are in equilibrium with our inner selves, envy can be a valuable guide, leading us to the things that are right for us.

I have treated many people whose envy led them into a more challenging and satisfying life. Ron came to me because he had overheard his girlfriend, a popular lecturer, making financial arrangements for a presentation she had been invited to give at a national conference. When he heard that the organizers were going to pay her six hundred dollars and cover all her expenses, he became upset and envious. He told her, "You mean to tell me that you are getting all that money and a free trip just to talk for one hour? Do you know how hard I have to work to make that kind of money?"

After doing a few *pláticas* and *limpias* with me, Ron realized that what he envied in his girlfriend—her ability to talk in front of large groups of people—was something that he desired for his own life. He realized that he was a very extroverted, charismatic person stuck in a job that was frustrating to him. Although he had many talents, he had never really done anything with them. He periodically decided to go back to college and finish his degree, but each time he quit after taking only a few courses. Ron had the ability to do what he envied in his girlfriend, but he wasn't doing anything about it. Instead of acting, he was reacting.

Many times people with envy make halfhearted attempts to obtain the object of their desire, but don't have the energy inside to make them really happen. As Ron and I worked together, I helped him gather that energy and focus it on something. Although he didn't go back to college, he started speaking in public by becoming an advocate for a homeless organization for which he was doing volunteer work. The feeling of using his energy and talents to be of service to others gave Ron a strong sense of self-esteem and satisfaction.

Envy Among Family Members

Envy among family members is very common, yet this feeling is largely ignored in our culture. Parents often unconsciously set up envious relationships between siblings by having a favorite child who gets more attention than the others. In large families, children can feel envy if they sense that there is not enough love to go around, or if they feel that a brother or sister is getting more attention than they are. One of my clients was the youngest of five children. By the time she was born, she felt that her mother was just too worn out and distracted to give her enough love and attention. An older sister tried to mother her, but it never felt like enough.

The root of envy among siblings can sometimes be a bad relationship between the parents. Even though it is true that scarcity is often at the root of envy, I have also seen a lot of people from very poor families who were rich in love because their mother and father loved each other and their children dearly. Often a husband or wife who does not feel as if he or she is getting enough love and support from a spouse will make a son or daughter a surrogate partner. Sometimes a child will have a close relationship with one parent, but will envy the sibling who has a close relationship with the other parent. This is fertile ground for the spreading of gossip. A daughter will go up to her mother and say, "Do you know that your darling little boy is going out and getting drunk every night?" Or the son will say, "Do you realize that your darling little girl is getting it on in the backseat of her boyfriend's car every weekend?" Things become worse when someone tells you a story and asks you not to repeat it; for example, when a parent says, "You are my favorite child, but don't tell your sister," all kinds of unbalanced and hurtful energy dynamics are created.

When my father became sick and had to go into the hospital shortly after my mother died, I experienced a rush of strong emotions and panic. Even though I was in my thirties, I felt fearful that my father would die and leave me without any parents. Picking up some gifts and flowers for him, I rushed to his hospital room. I cried and cried, saying, "Please, Daddy, don't die. If you do, I'll be an orphan. I love you, I love you." I must have told him I loved him a hundred times.

Wide-eyed at my passionate outpouring of grief, he said, "*Mijita*, I'm not that sick. Why are you so upset?"

I told him, "Well, Mom died a few months ago, and it occurred to me that I could lose both my parents. It scared me." We spent a beautiful afternoon together. He told me many things about himself and about Mom and how much he cared for her. We felt very close to each other. When I was leaving, I gave him a big hug and told him several times, "I love you, Daddy. I love you." He told me, "I love you too."

That's when it hit me that all these years I had been longing to hear him say those words. I had always known that he loved me, but I had wanted to hear him say it out loud, to hear that melody. I danced all the way home.

Being who I am, I had to share this news with my sisters. I called Rosario first. "I went to see Dad, and he told me he loved me," I told her, babbling on and on about how happy I was. At that point there was a long painful pause at the other end of the telephone wires, and I felt the pain, tension, and envy come toward me as a palpable wave. Slowly, weakly, and hesitantly, Rosario said, "Well . . . he's never told *me* that he loves me."

I was overwhelmed with a feeling of sadness and hopelessness. My first thought was, "What's the use? I can't really keep my happiness. My happiness makes other people sad." But then, Divine Energy came through me, and it occurred to me to say, "Go buy him some flowers and gifts, rush into his room hysterically crying, and tell him a hundred times over, 'I love you, Daddy. Please don't die.' And he'll tell you that he loves you too. In other words, *Chayito*, work for it like I did."

Gossip and Spreading Rumors

Gossip and spreading rumors are directly related to envy. What is worse, the person who starts the rumor is usually a friend, family member, or co-worker of the object of the gossip. After all, people have little interest in gossiping about those whom they don't know. Many times I have seen the shock and betrayal on the faces of clients who come to see me because a friend, lover, or family member who envies them has started some kind of hurtful rumor about them. Betrayal is one of the most painful emotions that humans can feel when we discover that the person who has done us wrong is someone for whom we care. It destroys our trust in love, the thing we humans desire most in life.

A fifteen-year-old teenager named Julia was brought to see me by her parents because she refused to go to school.

They were worried about her because she was becoming withdrawn and sad.

The first thing I noticed about Julia was her inner glow. She was a beautiful young woman with smooth ivory skin, small even features, and a spiritual strength that lit up her delicate face. Julia was upset because she had found out that a close friend at school had heard her throw up in the bathroom, and had begun spreading rumors that Julia was losing weight because she was suffering from bulimia. The friend had done this in retaliation when a boy that she had a crush on asked Julia out instead of her. Since these rumors had spread throughout the school, Julia was too embarrassed to go back. She felt a deep sense of betrayal at what her friend had done.

In reality, Julia had a chronic kidney disease. The new medication she was taking made her nauseous and contributed to her weight loss. Because she was very shy, she did not like to talk about her illness. A short time after I worked with her, she was able to end her relationship with her friend, and write an article in the school newspaper about living with a kidney disease. She received tremendous support from her peers, and in treatment she learned about the destructive power of envy. She is now doing well in school and her health has improved. Recently she even called me up and interviewed me for an article she is writing for the school newspaper on how curanderismo treats envy. She is taking care of herself and others at the same time.

One aspect of envy that Julia's story makes clear is the if-I-can't-have-it-you-can't-either syndrome. We can often become crafty and sophisticated in the way that we undermine others. Sometimes we do it virtuously: "I don't like to judge, but . . ." A common form of gossip in the workplace designed to undermine the competition subtly is "Please don't reveal the source of this, because I don't like to harm anyone, but did you know that So-and-so did such-and-such?"

When We Are Envied by Others

There is an old Spanish proverb that says, *"Vale más causar envídia que no lástima,"* "It is better to be envied than pitied." Let's face it, most people, if given a choice, would prefer to be the object of envy than the person who is pining away after something that he or she doesn't have. Knowing that we are envied might even fill us with a sense of superiority. But if we don't have a strong sense of self, another person's envy has the potential to make us sick. Some of us, like Nancy Kerrigan, can become very real physical victims of envy.

A client of mine, a slim attractive Chicana woman in her forties, learned firsthand about the power of envy. Anna had long, beautiful, wavy hair that hung down to her waist and made her look gorgeous. A successful educator, she came to me because she wanted to work on a childhood trauma that had damaged her ability to trust in her strong power of intuition. Anna received many compliments about her hair, especially from men. Of course, she knew just how to run her fingers through it so that you couldn't help but admire it.

The next time I saw her, I couldn't believe my eyes. The hair that she had been so proud of was dry, frizzy, and much, much shorter. She told me that a girlfriend of hers had suggested that she perm the top part of her hair because it was a little too straight and did not go with the more wavy bottom part. She looked in the mirror after her friend left, and her hair didn't look quite as good anymore, so she decided that her friend was right and that she should give herself a permanent. While she was working the solution into the top part of her hair, however, some of it dripped onto the wavy part, which made it go straight. Because the chemicals were so strong, they dried her hair and made it strawlike.

Anna was in shock. Her intuition had told her to leave her hair alone but she had not listened. Instead she had given in to the temptation to try making her hair even more beautiful than it already was. Now she had tight curls on top, while the rest was limp and dry. She ended up cutting her hair in an attempt to fix it, and it looked terrible.

One of the *limpias* we did together had a profound effect on her. She had saved the hair that she cut off, and she brought that to the ceremony. Anna had it tied with a beautiful ribbon, and we arranged it in the west, the place of letting go. We put a heart-shaped circle of cornmeal around it. In the east, we put a picture of her as a baby. She had been nicknamed *Peloncita,* which meant "little bald one." For her, this picture symbolized a new beginning. In the north, she placed a picture of her favorite grandmother, who had been a *sobadora.* This grandmother had passed on when Anna was a teenager, and Anna looked toward her for strength. She wanted to go beyond her outer experience, and she felt as if she needed a grandmother's wisdom and spirituality to find out what was really important in her life.

In the south, Anna placed pictures of herself at various ages while she was growing up. Each of these pictures represented a trauma, a time when she had lost her intuition. These were symbols of the *justos* that had made her give up her power. Finally she placed a picture of her friend in the west, along with the hair she had saved, because she felt that she needed to release that friendship. Honoring the intuition that was telling her that it was better for her to let that relationship go, Anna was able to release it with love. In the fifth direction we put a circle of cornmeal, symbolizing that Anna needed a strong community to validate who she was.

We made the journey through the five directions, and Anna said her prayers and stated her intentions. By the end of the ceremony, Anna realized that she had learned something valuable from the experience, that what she really wanted in life was to have a strong sense of her core inner self. In a sense, her friend actually helped her by finally letting Anna see that she was putting too much emphasis on her external appearance. "I realized that the compliments I had been receiving for my hair had made me focus too much on my outward beauty. If my hair was beautiful, maybe I could make it even more beautiful." By losing something that she really valued, Anna also learned the importance of not going against her intuition.

It took many months for Anna's hair to become healthy again, but she had learned a valuable lesson about the power of envy.

"I Just Can't Get Ahead"

One of the things that I often hear from the clients who come to see me is "I just can't get ahead because of all the people who envy me." While sometimes it is true that envy makes our path harder, often people are just using envy as an excuse to cover up what is really troubling them. Whether their complaints are legitimate or not, what these people need to do is to learn to empower themselves.

One of my clients, a fifty-year-old accountant, husband, and father named Juan, came to see me requesting a *limpia* because he was very angry with a co-worker. Juan was positive that he had been passed over for a promotion he wanted very badly because a co-worker had started a rumor that he was an alcoholic. He told me, "This guy's been envying me for a long time because I am better at my job than he is. What bothers me the most is how hypocritical he is. He pretended to be my friend, but then talked about me behind my back. I feel like a fool for trusting him. Now I hate the thought of going to work every day because I know the people in my office are talking about me. I feel like my reputation is ruined, but I can't afford to quit."

After a series of *limpias* and *pláticas*, Juan was able to take more responsibility for his situation. He began to realize that he had been too passive in his relationships at work, and decided to talk to his boss about his belief that this co-worker had spread false rumors about him. His boss admitted that he had heard the rumors, but told Juan that he knew he was not an alcoholic. Most important, he pointed out several specific reasons why Juan had not gotten the promotion. At the same time, he reassured Juan that he was very happy with his work and offered suggestions to help him improve his overall performance.

Juan also confronted his co-worker with the rumors. They did not heal their friendship, but the gossip stopped. Through accepting responsibility for his own passive patterns of behavior instead of blaming the envious attitude of a co-worker for his problems, Juan was able to heal the part of him that was keeping him from being assertive enough to get what he wanted.

The Person Who Envies

"Everything I have done, I have done for the wrong reasons," cried Cristina, a fifty-year-old lawyer and mother of two children. "I went to law school to meet the right husband. I had children because I was supposed to. I stay in my bad marriage because a divorce would make me look bad. Even though I hate the pressure and competition of my job, and I often get into rages with my secretary and the other lawyers in the firm, I am afraid to quit because of how it will look to other people. I feel like I have no identity—just a lot of masks that I take on and off all day."

When I first began working with Cristina, she felt that she could barely go on living because life was just too hard. She had just been diagnosed with breast cancer and was contemplating suicide because she "didn't want to be a burden" on her family. She also suffered from an anxiety disorder, high blood pressure, and high cholesterol. She was a perfectionist who didn't know how to relax, and I was her last hope.

Cristina had given her soul to her law practice, to the Porsche she drove, to her fancy house in the right neighborhood, and to the two hours she spent in the gym every day in order to look good. She had no hobbies and had little time to explore developing interests because she was a workaholic and spent twelve hours a day at her job. She was consumed by envy of all the people she saw who seemed happier than she was. She envied women who were artistic because she saw them as free spirits. She envied housewives because they could stay at home and be good wives and mothers. Because her marriage was a failure, she envied couples who had successful marriages because they looked so happy and content. She envied men because they "had it easier," she envied young women because she was getting "ugly and old," and she envied old women because she felt that, due to the cancer, she was going to die before she had a chance to retire and enjoy life.

Cristina's heart was twisted. When she came to see me, she did not realize that her problem was envy, but it soon became clear that envy was devouring her entire life. She was so afraid of dying that she had decided simply to kill herself and get it over with. Even greater than her fear of death was her fear of never having had a life at all. That is why she envied everyone around her whose life seemed more fun, fulfilling, and substantial than hers.

While we worked together I discovered that Cristina's father had been a very ambitious, hard-driving man who would do anything to get ahead. He had always wanted to go to college, and he had always wanted a son. As the oldest of three girls, Cristina became his surrogate son, and she and her father had a very close relationship. Since Cristina was very smart, ever since she could remember she had been told that she was going to college, and she fulfilled that ambition of her father's.

Cristina saw her mother as weak, passive, and ineffective,

and did not want to be like her at all. This poor image of her mother that she carried around inside made it hard for her to connect with the powerful feminine part of her soul.

She no longer loved her husband, who was also a professional, but she was very attached to all of the material possessions that they shared together. Every time she thought about divorce, she became frightened about whether or not she could make it on her own, and how she could live without all the "goodies" her marriage afforded her.

After we had worked together for a while, it became clear to me that Cristina really wanted to have a less demanding job that would allow her to spend more time at home and more time with outside hobbies and activities that would bring her pleasure. When I suggested this idea to her, she became terrified. Even though she knew on one level that she was living her father's life, she could not let go of that role for fear of angering him. She was also very attached to the prestige of being an attorney. Taking a less demanding job meant that she would have to trade off some of her professional status in the world.

The last *limpia* that we did together reflected her need to cut through her ambiguity. Her intent was to come to a decision either to stay with her old life or really choose to live. During the ceremony, it became very clear to me that Cristina wanted to maintain the status quo. All of her prayers involved asking God to help her to be happy with her husband, and help her to be content with her job. She just couldn't choose a different, more fulfilling kind of life for herself. This was the last time I saw her. Two years later, I saw in the obituaries that she had died of breast cancer.

Not everyone can be healed. Some people are just too damaged. To me, it felt as if Cristina just had too much leather around her soul. She was too deeply involved in living out the ambitions of her father and being a tough, macha woman. She never really had her life. Instead she chose to live with the burden of her envy.

Healing the Root of Envy

If a person has a relatively strong soul and spirit, she can heal the envy within herself. One way of doing this is simply to go to the person you envy and admit this to him or her. The honesty and sincerity of that action breaks the tension that is building and changes the energy between the two of you in an important way. If your friend wins the lottery, have the courage to go up to her and say, "You know, I really want to be happy for you but I'm not. When I think of you having all that money, I feel envious." It's actually good to say these words. When we say something like this, it breaks the intrusive connection that we build with people when we send them negative or envious thoughts. Admitting you are envious opens the door for incredible healing and strengthening of the friendship. This allows the person who is envious to get in touch with her shame, and this can often elicit very sympathetic, comforting behavior from the person being envied.

Sometimes envy can be a very humorous experience. Ever since I began thinking about writing my own book, I have been envious of well-known Chicana writers. I felt the "twisted heart" every time I heard that Demitria Martinez or Ana Castillo had a new book out. Last month I was doing a workshop in Las Cruces, New Mexico, for the Border Book

Festival. My workshop, called Weeping Soul and Twisted Heart: A Curandera Heals with Poetry, combined my own poetry with concepts found in curanderismo. I talked about how creative and spiritual aspects of our selves are unearthed when we heal the envy and soul loss in our hearts. As an example of envy, I told the audience of over one hundred fifty people how my own envy of Ana Castillo had twisted my heart and how writing my book had helped to heal me. After I had mentioned her name twice, I noticed a hand go up in the audience. It was Ana Castillo! I was busted. I had confessed my envy to her in person without even knowing it. This was both a funny and embarrassing moment for me. Her question was, "Elena, since you mentioned my name twice, how do I protect myself from envious people like you?" The audience howled and I was humbled. After my talk she came up to me and we hugged. Healer heal thyself.

When I have admitted to someone that I am envious, I have often found that it is a great relief to release the shame of that envy and heal it. Sometimes myself or the other person will shed tears. This almost always offers you both a chance to become closer.

A logical worry that we all carry is, "What if I tell a person, 'I'm envious of you. I wish I could be happy about your good fortune and I'm not' and he says, 'Well, fuck you'"? I can say with confidence that the situation doesn't usually go this way. We all know deep inside that we have been envious of someone at one time or another, so when someone approaches us with sincerity and confesses envy, we can easily identify with his or her feelings. There is something touching about people's vulnerability at such times, and their fear. When I give lectures on envy and talk about admitting it, I often get a kick out of how people often come up to me afterward and practice admitting their envy. They might say something like, "I envy you your long hair," or "I wish I could give a lecture that makes people laugh the way that you do."

Another humorous experience I had with envy recently occurred while I was visiting my sister. My mother had some poetry books from Mexico that were her treasures. She kept them in a special box, and we children were never supposed to touch them. Years later, after she had died, I discovered that my sister Irma had taken the books and was keeping them in her home. Since I had always wanted to be a writer and had been fascinated with the books as a little girl, I felt crushed and full of envy. All my feelings of being the little sister who always got the hand-me-downs came rushing back to me.

"You got Mom's books?!!" I shouted.

"Oh, give me a break, your name is all over the fucking books," she said.

"What?" I said, shocked.

"Come over here and look."

Sure enough, I had written my name all over these books. I had totally forgotten. After each poem in the table of contents, I had written "*la famosa* Elena Martinez," or "*la hermosa* (most beautiful) Elena Martinez." I had also included the date and the fact that I was eleven years old, so I knew exactly when I had crossed the boundary and written all over my mother's precious books.

This was a very healing experience for both myself and my sister. I said, "Okay, fine, you can keep the books. I've already put my mark on them." We laughed and laughed, and our envy was healed. When you are close to somebody, admitting envy doesn't have to be a scary experience.

If you don't have the courage to talk to someone face-to-face, or if you feel that there are important reasons why you shouldn't talk to him or her, you can admit to yourself that you are envious and take your own steps to heal it. You can put yourself in a meditative state and admit that anger to yourself, and then ask yourself what the anger is trying to say about you. How important to you is having that thing that you are coveting? Do you really want it, or is it just a whim? If you are coveting a size 8 butt, are you really able to eat tiny portions of food for the rest of your life? Are you willing to put in three hardworking years to get your Ph.D.? Do you really want to move to Hawaii? Sometimes envious feelings are just whims, and you need to ask your heart, "What is it that you really want?" When we admit to ourselves that we feel envy, we can use these feelings as a mirror for change.

If your envy doesn't go away, but begins to eat away at your heart and soul, then you need a curandera. Depending on how much your soul has been injured, you might just need a *plática* and a *limpia*, or you might actually need a soul retrieval. Polito, the man I spoke about at the beginning of this chapter, fell into the latter category because his wounds ran very deep. During one of the *pláticas* I did with him, he drew a picture of his family, but he did not put himself into the picture. All of the other family members were very separate from one another. This helped show me the intensity of his feelings of separation from his family, and shed light on the intense envy Polito felt toward people who had close families, marriages, and friendships.

After giving him several *pláticas* and *limpias* to identify his lost soul parts, we did our first soul retrieval. I put Polito into a trance and told him that I was going to send him on a shamanic journey to find a lost part of his soul. I drummed for quite a while and, when I felt his journey coming naturally to an end, I helped him come back out of his trance state. Then I asked him gently, "Polito, what did you see? Did you find your soul?"

He started to weep, telling me, "I saw a child, a very small child who was reaching out toward me with his little arms." In illustration Polito reached out plaintively with his arms, "But he had no head because everybody else always does his thinking for him. This child had blood dripping from his arms, legs, and chest. He said, 'I have been wounded so many times.' Right before you stopped the drumming, I saw a lightning rod that said, 'Wake up!'"

During the next soul retrieval, Polito saw himself as a little boy again. His head and shoulders were bent and he was looking down at the ground. He was hiding outside because his mom and dad were inside the house getting drunk. The little boy told Polito that he wanted to be happy but that his parents were drunk and would not listen to him. He felt so unwanted.

Afterward, while we were talking, Polito told me that he used to go outside and hide for hours. He had always been envious of his brother Juan because he was his mom's favorite child. Many feelings began to surface, and he told me that he wondered what his life would be like if his father had not died. He started to cry, and said, "I wish my father was still with me."

Polito did overcome a good part of his envy of families and closeness by going back to his cultural roots. He began to attend some of the Pueblo Indian fiestas and dances, which gave him a greater sense of cultural identity and a sense of belonging somewhere. His depression began to lift. He had never known his grandparents, because they had died when he was very small, but he was comforted when I told him, "The earth that we walk on is the ashes of our grandparents."

The Child in the Moon

Many of the clients that I treat for *envidia* and other types of soul loss see their lost soul parts as a small, lonely, and neglected child. One of the most frequent images that I see when I go on trance journeys to find the souls of my clients is a child huddled on the moon. This child is often wild looking, with matted hair, skin encrusted with dirt, and soiled pants. Often when I call to it and ask it to come with me, it will not respond right away, and I have to befriend it patiently. At these times, I never rush the child, but tell myself that I have as much time as I need to win its trust. I would never make it go with me forcibly. That would be a violation of the soul's essence.

First I ask the child if I can comb its hair. It lets me do so for a little while, then runs away. When it comes back, I ask it if I can take it to the river and bathe it, which I do very tenderly because its skin is so fragile and has been hurt so much. The purpose of doing these things with the child is not to clean it up and make it into some kind of presentable, ideal child but simply to win its trust, to treat gently the energy that has gone into hiding because of pain and trauma. When the child is finally ready to come back to me, I take it into my arms, and we fly together back to Earth where I blow its little spirit back into the top of my client's head. The child in the moon may be filthy and wild, but it has valuable energy that we need in order to live. We must learn to love that child unconditionally and reintegrate it back into ourselves.

Envy is a secret and shameful emotion, but it is also a valuable one. When a part of our soul is missing, and we are envying the energy, talents, and accomplishments of others, we can see more clearly what parts of ourselves we need to reclaim. We need to bring back the child in the moon, to use envy as a mirror to tell us what our soul wants and who we really are.

Getting people to admit *envidia* is the hardest part of my job. It helps when I tell clients, "We all feel envy because this is a part of being human." We need to transform our envy into self-love, embracing that injured little child and integrating it back into our beings, even if the stitches on our soul give us occasional pain. We need to reintegrate all parts of us, even the parts that seem wild, scary, dirty, and unattractive, back into the whole. Unless we can do this, we will never really have the ability to live up to our true capacity, and to experience our fullest capacity for love. When I do my work, I often pray to the Aztec cosmic mother, Coyolxauhqui:

> *Mother that glows in the dark, help me*
> *ride this weird energy mine until your*
> *luminous, magnetic heart transforms me*
> *into love. For I truly want to love. Truly.*

Chapter Six

Apprenticeship
Student Teacher, Teacher Student

For every teacher, there comes a time when she wants to pass on her long years of knowledge and experience to others. After nearly two decades of studying and practicing curanderismo, that time finally came for me. I had started teaching curanderismo long before I took on formal apprentices. I really began when I was working as a nurse in El Paso, Texas, a town with a large Chicano population, right next to the Mexican border. During the seventies, it became very popular in the medical field to practice cross-cultural medicine, a medicine that recognized and respected each patient's cultural values and beliefs. In a very real sense, I was thrown into talking about curanderismo because the push toward learning cross-cultural nursing was so great, and the people who could really talk about it so few. I was often asked to give lectures or presentations on folk beliefs and folk diseases and their cures. For many people, this was their *only* source of information on curanderismo because there was so little published material about it. What existed were mainly dry academic articles written by scholars with preconceived notions about how primitive this medicine was.

That's not to say that I had all the answers. In the beginning, I often knew just a little bit more than my audience. But the hunger for information was so great that people did not care. During this period, I was traveling across the border to Juárez, Mexico, to work with curanderas there. I'd learn a little bit, and then come back and share what I'd found out. People in my audiences would ask me questions and I would answer them to the best of my ability. If I honestly didn't know the answer, I'd say so, and then go back to Mexico to find someone who did know. When I look back on that time, I'm astonished at how willing people were to listen to someone who knew as little as I did. I also realize that, if I had been an Anglo woman, I would have been shot down immediately—"Oh, what does she know!" But because of my brown skin, my parents who had been born in Mexico, my Mayan ancestry, and my grandmother who had been a curandera, people were willing to listen to me and to trust what I had to say. In this way, I was able to take the time to grow into a good teacher and lecturer who *did* have some knowledge to share.

By the late eighties, I had become a national speaker who traveled regularly to many states and met with other health-care professionals. These individuals began asking me if I gave workshops in curanderismo. To my surprise, I realized that these modern medical practitioners didn't just want to study curanderismo, they wanted to become curanderas. One of the things that they wanted to learn was how to do *limpias*, so I thought, why not take them to a very beautiful place in nature, Ghost Ranch, and give them a workshop? I taught these weekend intensives from Friday to Sunday, twice a year, for five years.

I began by teaching participants some very basic things: the symbolism of the altar and how to set one up, the meaning of the five sacred directions, how to do ceremony and ritual using the directions as a foundation. The only way I could think of to show the group how to do *limpias* and soul retrievals was to have them practice on each other. Breaking them down into pairs, I taught them how to listen, how to elicit information, and how to help a client really focus on what he wants to release during the *limpia*. Often this meant encouraging the psychologist or therapist conducting the *plática* to let go of preconceived assumptions and rules of interaction related to a particular field of psychology and to follow her deep intuition.

I was amazed at what came out of these doctors, nurses, therapists, and social workers—all kinds of physical and sexual abuse, trauma after trauma. Most of all, I noticed how common themes began to emerge among these health-care professionals. All of them had to manage so many responsibilities every day, help so many people, witness so much suffering. Because they had to give so much, their own wounds had gone untended for years and years. Many of them talked about how tired they were. In a very real sense, the gatherings at Ghost Ranch began to turn into healer-heal-thyself workshops.

I knew that I couldn't do this teaching alone, so I always brought a couple of assistants with me. My sister Irma Martinez, who is also an accomplished curandera, was a frequent helper, as was my friend Linda Velarde, who is an incredible healer.

Even with their support, it took tremendous energy for me to keep thirty people aware, connected, and focused. I even went so far as to prepare essential oil mixtures and waters scented with herbs and essential oils, and keep them on the altar to rub or sprinkle on people when I saw that their spirits needed to be brought back to the room and to the task at hand.

After the *pláticas*, which took most of Friday, we would spend the evening doing drumming and chanting. I have always found sound to be a powerful healing tool because it awakens people's energy and connects them to their spirits. Drums are very effective in unlocking frozen feelings, and chanting opens the throat chakra, releasing petrified emotions. Our drumming and chanting sessions opened everyone up even more, allowing them further to release and transcend their traumas and sorrow.

The following morning, participants would tell me about the incredible lucid dreams they'd had the night before, and we would incorporate them into their healing. Then we would begin doing the *limpias*. I had set all the ingredients for the *limpia* up on the altar, the eggs, water, *romero*, and scented oils. I again divided the group into pairs and gave them basic instructions. Those beautiful experiences will be forever engraved in my heart. I will never forget the sounds of people healing, the pitiful crying and the laughing, the smell of copal and *romero*, and the sight of my assistants walking around that huge room, compassionately helping the participants wherever they were needed.

These *limpias* were a preparation for the group soul retrieval with which I always ended the weekend. I gave the students the afternoon off and suggested that they find a beautiful isolated place to sit and think about the part of themselves that they wanted to reclaim. The next day, everyone came back together and the group soul retrieval took place.

One of the things that I have always loved about doing group soul retrievals is that I never know what Spirit is going to ask of me. As time went on, and a core group of people, mostly women, began coming to every workshop, they became more and more experienced at understanding the process. Because of that, the soul retrievals became more elaborate, incorporating elements of theater and mystery. I was happy with this development because one of the things that I was really trying to teach the people who came to the workshop was not to get stuck in any particular procedure or form. What was more important was teaching them to get in touch with group energy, what the group needed.

People in the medical profession are often caught up in the idea of unalterable procedures and steps. Soul retrieval is not a recipe that comes out of a procedural manual. One of the things that I learned in Mexico was how too much structure can actually cause the soul to go into hiding. Our souls are experts at hiding anyway, and our job as healers is to catch the soul unawares. This is a very loving ambush. When people are really caught unawares, they show their true natures. I remember one story told to me by two friends who are lesbians. One of the women was always acting very strong and tough—a real *macha*. One evening, both of them returned home from a day trip. They were unaware that the brother of one woman had a key to the house and had let himself in to get something. As they reached the door, he swung it open. Neither woman could see who he was in the twilight, and both were startled. What was so comical, however, was that the macha panicked, pushing her lover into the doorway, and ran away. Startled, her true, timid soul showed itself.

Because we have so many masks, it is hard for the healer to get the soul to peak out so that she can say "Gotcha!" We must first see all parts of ourselves clearly if we are to heal.

The Wild Boar

I remember one particular soul retrieval in which I decided really to change things around. I felt that it was important to show the workshop participants how to allow the soul to tell us what it needs. For this soul retrieval, I planned to bring in the animal spirits in a more concrete way. We had already been doing this at earlier workshops with wooden and metal masks that I had purchased in Mexico and Peru, but I wanted to see if I could take everyone deeper. With this in mind, I had asked one of my assistants, Jeri, to prepare an animal costume and bring it to the workshop. She was to be the guiding spirit who went and got all of the participants and led them into the room where the four directions and the altar were set up.

Jeri had created a very elaborate wild boar costume and had spent much time practicing how to act, sound, and move like this wild animal. As my assistants and I prepared for the group soul retrieval that weekend, I began to get the feeling that Jeri really needed to learn something else. I felt that she had been intellectualizing too much about the place of the north and needed to get more deeply and emotionally in touch with her ancestors. So I asked another of my students to become the boar, and I asked Jeri to take on the persona of the north instead.

I wanted very much for the directions to come alive during this soul retrieval, so I placed a living manifestation of their energy at each point of the compass. In the west stood my comadre Linda, dressed in black with a skeleton mask. In our culture we call this figure La Huesuda (the Bony One). In Western culture she is known as the Grim Reaper. La Huesuda invites people to participate in the cycles of death and rebirth. I asked Jeri, the woman who would have been the boar, to become the Old Man, a stooped figure dressed in coveralls who greeted the workshop participants in the north. In the south was my sister Irma who dressed as a little girl with braids and freckles. I stood in the east, dressed as the goddess of the sun and of mystery.

By allowing the workshop participants to visit the living directions, I wanted to provide them with an opportunity to get more deeply in touch with their fears and their hopes and to open them up to their vulnerabilities. I wanted to move their assemblage point, that place within each of us that has certain fixed expectations and set beliefs, and I knew I could do that most effectively by bringing them face-to-face with the unexpected. To keep the mystery intact, I had all of them wait in a separate room until the ugly, snarling, obnoxious wild boar came to drag or lead them into the ritual room, one by one.

It was amazingly revealing how each of the participants reacted. Thrown off balance, they all began showing their true colors. Most were afraid, some simply surrendered, and all were nervous and uneasy. One woman was so fearful that she even began leading a revolution, trying to talk everyone into resisting when the wild boar came back for her next victim. "We just don't have to go with her. Why should we? We don't have to do this." Being shocked into confronting our hidden behaviors and feelings is a scary experience because we are all so fragile. When our masks are removed, often a sad, wounded child is uncovered. But, as I stress to my students, all parts of the self must be found and reintegrated if we are to learn to accept and love ourselves truly.

After each of the participants had visited the four living directions, they all lay down in a circle on the floor. When everyone was present, I took them through a shamanic journey in search of their lost souls.

At the end of the trance journey, we had a talking circle, giving everyone a chance to share his or her experiences. In a talking circle, everyone speaks from the heart, and everyone takes turns speaking until all has been said. Only the person holding the eagle feather, which is passed around the circle, may speak, and the rest must strive to be really present with what that person is saying, listening without interrupting or trying to "fix" the person who is doing the talking.

To give you a fuller idea of how this particular workshop (all women) was experienced by those who attended, and what they learned from it, I've asked three of the participants to share their stories. The first is told by Jeri, whom I asked to play the Old Man instead of the Wild Boar; the second by Soledad, who played the Wild Boar; and the third by Lorraine, who was a participant in the soul retrieval itself. These three extraordinary women later went on to become my apprentices.

Jeri: Surrendering and Becoming the Ancestor

"Several years ago Elena asked me if I would be willing to help at her workshops at Ghost Ranch. I had been participating in those workshops since the first Dance of the Curanderos in 1988. Over the years, as I gradually experienced my own healing, I was able to start giving back to Elena and the others. I began with basic physical chores, such as cleaning, gathering firewood, and moving furniture. As I learned more, I was asked to do more—preparing the fire pit, cleansing the dance circle, and eventually working with Elena and the other curanderas in their planning circle.

"I was so proud and anxious when she called and directed me to bring the trappings of an animal, a wild, fierce animal. I was to be the Beast in the soul retrieval of the entire community. I got to work—praying for guidance, going into the wilderness to unlock the imagery of this part of the spirit. At the same time I was working on recognizing my own masks, the illusions I have created to cover myself.

"As the ceremonies [leading up to the soul retrieval] progressed, I was content and comfortable doing familiar tasks, but it became obvious that this time was different. Nothing I did was quite right. The chairs needed to be moved again, my ideas were lightly passed over. When I was asked to gather wooden staffs for each *maestra*, I thought, 'Surely I can do this.' Into the rain and down the arroyo I went and found beautiful, smooth, and strong staffs. Feeling like a child, I lovingly presented my gifts. 'Oh, no, this one just isn't quite right. It's not what I wanted. Actually, none of these are. You can take them back.' My mask smiled, and I said, 'Okay.'

"Rain and tears drew me back down the arroyo. I lay on the dirt and I cried. I wasn't worthy. My worst fears bared my face and I saw the Beast. I felt frozen, numb with fear.

"I returned and dressed in white for the *limpias*. My comadre Luisa and I sat expectantly in the circle, ready for the work to begin, little realizing we were in its grasp already. 'No, no, Luisa and Jeri, I want you to receive the *limpia* this time.' I looked at Luisa and her eyes were round and dark. I thought, I could fall into them, but I can't move. I've become stone, hard white stone. But something deep inside was moving, and it was warm. It was growing and telling me it was time to surrender, and I knew I had to. Somehow, Irma was with me, holding me, reassuring me that surrender and death are not final, rocking me in her arms. Somehow I knew I was being tested by Elena, by the comadres, by myself. I felt myself dying into the earth. Warmth, love, singing, returning, surrender, belonging, peace—all flooded me.

"Later, as we began preparation for the soul retrieval,

Elena said, 'I want you to give your Beast to Soledad. She's to be the Beast.' The *limpia* had left me prepared and stripped clean of my own harsh voice, my self-doubt, down to the bone. 'I want you to be the *Viejo*,' Elena said. I was ready, I would be this. She put the lines of age on my face and I saw clearly through her stern look. Her mask was transparent when she said, 'You know this has all been a test!' I was laughing and crying with the love bursting out. 'Yes,' I whispered, 'I know this.' Walking across the field I began to experience the change. My walking stick and my cigarette seemed an extension of my worn hand. My body grew lighter. It bent and my head bowed to watch the ground. My feet shuffled. Can this be me?

"I surrendered and took Irma's arm for help. She was so beautiful and radiant. I remembered being in the north, the place of the ancestors. I was there, but my body was transformed. So many voices were behind me in the north. I surrendered and they came into me. Each talked to their children, my comadres, as they were presented to me for a blessing.

"Afterward, Elena suggested I go rest. 'Look at your face,' she said, 'you have surrendered your masks.' I went alone to my room, lit a candle, and looked into the mirror. I was transformed. I saw the eyes, the face, the spirit, the soul, the healer, the student, the teacher, the ancient one, the child, and the Beast. They were all me."

Soledad: Becoming the Beast

"At the first workshop I attended at Ghost Ranch I was hurting a lot, in need of a *limpia*, confused, looking for answers. By the second workshop, I had done a lot of work in my personal life. I was more at peace, open to change, waiting for a challenge. Elena perceived this. On the third afternoon as we were going to dinner, she approached me and told me I was going to be part of the soul retrieval. I was to act as the nagual (a person who can transform into an animal form, or can summon their own animal guides or spirits). The *Nagual* or Beast form I was to take would be that of a Wild Boar. It didn't occur to me to resist or question. I had learned that lesson long ago from Elena. I knew that she was moving my assemblage point, that she had a plan, and that I needed to follow it without question.

"Another comadre, Jeri, had made an elaborate costume for the Boar. It didn't occur to me at the time that she had made it for herself. It was a beautiful leather covering that fit like a toga. Jeri had made hand pieces out of bark that were to be wrapped around my hands with leather straps. A hideous Boar mask completely covered my head and shoulders.

"There were five of us, one woman for each of the five directions. Each person dressed accordingly and each had her role to perform. It was my task to bring the twenty women into the room and lead them to each of the four directions, then lead them to the middle of the room where they would lie down. All of this took place in a large darkened room already filled with the power, mystery, cleansing, and Spirit of the work we had done for the past three days.

"Elena told me that it was my job to move the assemblage point for each woman—to startle them and catch the soul off guard, so that it might speak. She didn't tell me how to do this, she just said, 'Trust your intuition, comadre, you'll know what to do. But be ruthless with them. You may need to be rough. Push them, wake them up, bring that soul to the surface.'

"We prepared right after dinner for perhaps two hours. We combed our hair, and those who required makeup took great care to get it right. We all helped each other. We even painted our toe- and fingernails bright red. Elena explained that everything mattered, every detail, every word, every gesture, from this point on.

"It is believed that by putting on the costume of an animal, a curandera or shaman can become a nagual. It certainly felt that way to me. I put on the leather covering, the bark hand pieces, and, finally, the mask. I was the Boar.

"The women were waiting for us. I knew that I had to be aggressive, ruthless, frightening. I felt myself hunch over, arms dangling, knees slightly bent. I let out a low muffled snort, then another, then a growl. I moved to the door of the waiting room and then I began to pound and kick at it, using my shoulder to ram against the wood. I heard the first startled screams and laughs come from the room. This egged me on. Growling, I opened the door, and saw the women sitting close to one another. I shuffled quickly through them, stepping on feet and bumping people out of the way, grabbed someone by the arm, and began dragging her into the outer room.

"I slammed the door behind me and gave the woman a firm shove toward the first direction, forcing her to kneel in front of the Old Man of the north. I then led my victim to each of the other three directions, growling and pushing her when it was necessary.

"At the end of the fourth direction, I led the woman to the center and made her lie down. There she had to wait in silence as I brought in each of the other women, one by one, growl after growl, battle after battle. I raged and so did they. At times the room would be silent with a fear that I could almost smell when I entered. I could feel women moving to the corners, trying to find safety. There were other times when I came upon a woman who completely transformed my demeanor. I could feel that woman embracing the fear. By doing so, she would dissolve my anger. I became a gentle, loving escort at those times instead of an intruder.

"This continued for, I believe, about three hours, but I lost all track of time. I just knew there were more women, they seemed to be multiplying. There were times when I grew tired, exhausted. I would enter the room looking for energy to replace mine. I would find that woman who was accepting of what was to happen. I would take her gently by the arm and she would comfort me. At long last, the final woman to be retrieved faced me alone in the dark, empty room. Exhausted, beaten down by my own force and anger, I walked calmly to her, extended an arm, bowed, and led her to the first direction.

"I drummed, made noise, and danced around the circle as the actual soul retrieval began. Elena began to take the women on their journey, and I, in my own way, followed them. There were sounds of laughter, crying, sobbing, and moaning. But unlike the muffled and restrained sounds in the room of terror, they were sounds of release and delivery.

"I was completely exhausted, spent, and immobile for a long while afterward. I had growled, grunted, hunched, and tormented for three hours. I never realized that being the aggressor took so much energy, was so draining and such a terrible burden. It was such a gift to have been given this role. I understood for the first time the fear of the aggressor, the helplessness, the loneliness, the confusion, and the inexplicable inability to stop. I felt the terrifying need to continue and the sad feelings of remorse, as though I could not stop the aggression, as if it had me, not I it. Being the Boar gave me the knowledge I needed to forgive my abusers, to see their hurt, their pain, their damage. Being the Boar gave me freedom from my own hatred and anger. It was my own soul retrieval."

Lorraine: In the Hands of the Wild Boar

"At this workshop, it took us two days to work up to where each one of us could focus on our own individual problems and eventually have an enlightening *limpia*. Most of the twenty women who attended this gathering had already taken one or two workshops, so we thought we were pretty well versed as to what to expect. Ha! Boy, did Elena have a surprise for us! She instructed us to dress up in our most festive, expressive clothing and had us gather in a foyer, just outside of the main room where the soul retrieval would take place.

"Excited about the tremendous insights we had been challenged with over the last two and a half days, we were chattering with each other, laughing and admiring each other's costumes, when suddenly, out from behind the door came a *tremendous* ROAR!!!! A sound so frightening that we all screamed at the top of our lungs. Along with the roar came the most frightening, ugly, hairy Boar. The Boar eventually came up to me, laid its paw on me, and dragged me into the room where the soul retrieval was to be held.

"I can honestly say that it was one of the most frightening times of my life. As I entered the darkened, misty room I became even more terrified as the Boar forced me to go to each direction, starting with the east. In the east stood a beautiful goddess representing the sun. 'Honor the east because it is the direction of the rising sun, it is the beginning of a new day for you.' She spoke with such mesmerizing and admirable authority that I actually began to cry, feeling all kinds of mixed feelings inside of me.

"The Boar then motioned for me to go over to the direction of the west where there was a ghostlike woman who said, 'You will let go. You will let your old self die.' At this point, I felt nothing but pure terror. I truly felt like running away. Although deep down inside I knew this was all a dramatic impersonation, I actually felt overwhelmed with intense emotion.

"The Boar then led me to the direction of the north, the place of our ancestors where a wise old grandfather stood with a hoe in his hand, large overalls, and a straw hat. At this point, I was overtaken with grief, respect, and veneration for this kindly old gentleman. In my mind's eye, I was looking at my father, my grandfather, my great-grandfather, and many more generations of ancestral grandfathers. He said, 'You will be all right, *mijita*, don't be afraid. I will always be there for you.' I cried with a very deep emotional love. I felt a powerful surge of pride for my ancestors, for the long line of generational strength and courage. These admirable attributes were actually a part of me. I thought, 'This is who and what I am.' All of the shame I'd ever had about myself and my ancestors disappeared, and I felt pride. I felt chills all over my body.

"The Boar, whom I no longer feared, led me to the direction of the south, the place of the child, the student, where there was a little girl playing hopscotch. She painted my cheeks with lipstick, and smiled and sang blissfully. Again, out poured the tears of joy and sadness. I saw the good, playful times of my childhood, as well as the scary, sad times.

"After I had completed the four directions, I was instructed to lie down in the center of the floor where I watched the Boar escort the rest of the twenty women to the four directions. It was an enlightening experience for me to see the various reactions. It made me realize that there are other options besides fear.

"Finally, we were led through an inner journey by Elena's gentle, soft voice. I visualized my inner soul and experienced a sweet, tranquil, loving journey that I will never forget, a journey that I often return to. I do not know what the other women experienced that particular weekend. I just know that our *maestra* Elena helped me to overcome the fear and shame that I had carried within me for several years. I was able to look fear straight in the eye. I've come to realize that I am a loving and spiritual woman and, with the help of the Creator, I want to eventually help others to have this realization about themselves."

From Teacher to Student

When I hear stories such as these, I am amazed at where teaching this work has taken me. As has happened so many times in my life, I begin with one idea and then it turns into something else. I started with the idea that I would teach something to a group of professionals, but they became my teachers. Through them, I learned how important it is to heal our wounds before we can heal the wounds of others. Before I began the workshops at Ghost Ranch, I had known, from my own experiences, how healing myself has helped me to become a better healer. But I only knew this from the personal level. After working with all of these health-care professionals, I learned this truth on a universal level. When I saw how terribly wounded many of these people were, I realized how deep our masks are. So many of the workshop participants were doctors, nurses, or people who ran big health-care agencies. On the surface, they looked so together, yet their poor souls were hurting so much. I admired the strength it took for each of them to admit that to themselves, and to heal. As they returned to later workshops, I could see how much they had progressed, how much they had applied what they had learned in their lives. I also admired their courage. They reminded me that no one is healed once and for all. Healing is a lifetime journey.

I cannot describe how profound it was to be in that beautiful setting, hearing people speak their truth, holding them in my arms while they went through their healing process. At the end of each workshop, no one wanted to go home. So many of them said to me, "This weekend, I learned for the first time what it felt like to be in a community that supported my sorrow and my healing and shared my joy, and I will miss that experience." As the years passed, the same people continued to come back, over and over, learning more and more, going deeper and deeper. As they returned, I was also able to go deeper in my commitment to discover what they really needed and to train them. Most of all, I was in awe of their commitment.

I began teaching these health-care professionals because I believed that they wanted to learn more about my culture so that they could serve the Hispanic population. Ultimately I realized that their commitment to this work came from a deep inner longing to heal themselves. Soul retrievals were one of the main keys to this process. Soon people at Ghost Ranch were humorously referring to me and my assistants as Ghost Busters because they saw us opening up all the musty closets of the soul and letting the ghosts out into the light of day. During those years, we all shared much sadness and pain, much laughter and joy.

Too Much Too Fast

Passing on the knowledge of curanderismo has not always been an easy journey. In my eagerness to share this medicine, I have sometimes made some profound mistakes. For many years, following the soul retrievals at Ghost Ranch, I gave each of my students a *sahumador* and a turkey feather so that they could do their own *limpias*. I even hired a potter here in Corrales, New Mexico, to specially make all of the *sahumadores*. One of the things that I soon learned was that you cannot give someone a sacred tool until he or she has the years of learning and depth of experience required to use it, and is really ready to receive it. Otherwise you will be disappointed by the lack of reverence that people bring to their tools. A *sahumador* represents your fire, the place where you are putting your energy while preparing to do a *limpia*. It is the vessel in which you burn your copal and make your sacred, purifying smoke.

Some of my students had broken their *sahumadores* within hours of receiving them, and asked me where they could pick up another one. For others, this gift triggered their self-importance and they began calling themselves curanderas and copying aspects of my workshops. I remember two students in particular who duplicated my workshop word for word. Ironically they left candles burning on the altar they had set up near an open window, and went out to lunch. The curtains caught fire and the room burned down.

When things like this happened, I always heard about them afterward. I soon began to realize that I had a responsibility as a teacher not to hand out information or tools to students without adequate preparation. Most important, I realized that I was opening people up too soon. They did not have the same kind of support system in their communities as I have here in New Mexico. Although I tried to do as much as I could by sending them encouraging letters, I had neither the time nor the energy to give them the ongoing support they needed. I was too far away and had too many other responsibilities, so these students were left without a mentor. When you give these kinds of workshops twice a year to twenty or twenty-five people, over time you end up with a huge group of people who are relying on you in one way or another.

Feeling overwhelmed, I began to ask myself, "What have I created?" Some of my students asked if they could come and live with me, and some did stay with me for a week or so. Many kept asking for more and more. Meanwhile, I had a son with mental retardation to watch over, a personal life to enjoy, and many local healing and teaching responsibilities. I began to realize that I needed to create some boundaries in my life. After teaching one of the weekend workshops at Ghost Ranch, I became so exhausted that it took me weeks to recover. Finally I stopped teaching at Ghost Ranch and took a break for two years to decide what was next for me. This was a painful time, because I missed those beautiful experiences, but I knew I needed a change of pace.

Taking on the First Apprentices

During this time, certain people were still coming to me and saying, "We want to learn more, we want to go deeper," so I began to think, "What if I try something new? What if I invite about twenty of the health-care professionals who have attended several workshops and have the true healing gift to work with me intensively, twice a month, for a year?" I asked about forty people to come for a potluck one Sunday afternoon to discuss this idea, figuring that about ten would show up. To my amazement, they all came—and brought their friends. My living room was overflowing.

The main question I asked prospective apprentices was,

"Do you have the strength to go through what it takes to become a curandera?" I wanted apprentices whom I could trust, to whom I could refer clients when I couldn't take care of all the people who called me for healing. I was looking for a true commitment. Learning curanderismo takes a lifetime, and I only wanted to train people who would represent it in a good and honorable way.

From the fifty people that showed up that afternoon, I chose twenty-three. It quickly became apparent that only nineteen had the dedication and a realistic idea of what was expected to be able to finish the training. One woman, who was a tarot card reader, felt as if she already knew about curanderismo because her mother was a curandera. She did not want to go through the necessary steps because she somehow thought that she had inherited all the knowledge that she needed. Even though some of the young women could remember sitting at the knee of a grandmother who was a curandera, learning incredible things, it was also true that they came from a generation where the knowledge was suppressed and not completely passed on. For example, although Alice, whose Nahuatl name is Ozomatl, shared beautiful memories of her *nene*, her paternal great-grandmother, who taught her where to lay her hands on people to help them heal, she knew that she still had much to learn before she could think of herself as a curandera.

It was obvious that about half of the women I chose to be my apprentices were more advanced than the others. They had already trained in alternative healing modalities such as Rolfing and massage therapy, knew much about giving *limpias*, and had already attended many of my workshops and lectures. For that reason, I divided the apprentices into beginner and advanced groups. Many interesting dynamics flowed out of this decision. Some people became very competitive, saying to themselves and others, "I'm in the advanced group." Ironically, I later discovered that some of the beginners quickly became more proficient than the advanced students. Although some of the advanced students had an incredible gift for curanderismo, they also had unresolved issues that kept them from progressing as quickly as others. The beginners, who were more willing to work on their issues, soon caught up to, and then even passed, the advanced students.

One thing I learned from this experience was that a person can never afford to stop growing. As I watched the transformations and soul-searching going on in my apprentices, I would sometimes feel as if I were looking at myself in a mirror. I would think, "There's me five years ago," or "There's something I was struggling with a month ago." Teaching my apprentices was, and continues to be, a humbling and enlightening experience.

I had gotten my training as a curandera the hard way, by having to go out and search for teachers and figure out many things for myself. I didn't want my apprentices to go through that struggle, to suffer and make the same mistakes that I had. I had longed for a good support system while I was training, and I often had to travel a long distance to be in the company of my peers. I knew that my apprentices could be a good support system for each other. Today, I can truly say with pride that they have become a family and support system for me as well as for each other. When one of us is ill, the others bring food to her. They bless each other's houses, and spend time with each other's families. Recently, when one of the women was leaving a job, four of my apprentices went to her house all by themselves and gave her a *limpia.* Hearing about this made me very happy. Before, they had always asked me to be present when they did this kind of work. Now they are taking care of themselves.

We always ended each of our bimonthly classes with a talking circle, and many issues came up, especially in the beginning. For example, there were originally only two men in the group, and some people wanted to know why there were only two. Some of the Chicanas wanted to know why there were white women in the group. In talking circles, they asked, "How can they become curanderas? This isn't their culture." I understood this question because I have suffered the same sort of racism and oppression that these women had, but I also knew that we have to move beyond that. When I asked each woman to become part of the group, I had not been looking at her skin color, but at her gift, her commitment to study this medicine. At the end of the year, however, I was gratified to hear one of the Chicanas tell the talking circle that her greatest teachers had been the white women in the group. I was relieved to hear this because I know that I cannot teach consciousness and awareness to a person. That is something that each person has to learn for herself.

I had not been expecting all of these issues to arise. I had an agenda and thought we would get right down to work. But in life, what we plan and what actually happens often turn out to be very different things. The most important lesson I learned from this experience was that there needed to be more talking circles because my apprentices had many issues to heal. As time went on, a great deal of healing did take place in these circles.

The Meaning of Apprenticeship

One of the big differences between my year-long training program for apprentices and the weekend workshops at Ghost Ranch is that the latter were only introductions, just a little taste of curanderismo. While tremendous healing and personal transformation went on during these weekends, those who attended them were not qualified to go out and be practicing curanderas. Since participants came from all over the U.S., many of them had no support system of alternative healers to go home to. One of the things that I have learned is that *no one* can be a healer without the support of the community. Because soul and spirit are incorporated within the work one does with the patient, because curanderismo does not separate the healer from the healed, this work brings up deep issues for both the client and the curandera—and sometimes this can be overwhelming for the healer. I truly believe that Niño Fidencia died at the age of thirty-two because he was completely worn out.

If I didn't have someone I could call up at the end of the day and say, "I am so exhausted, I just did four *limpias*,"—someone who really understood what that meant—I don't think I would be able to practice curanderismo for very long. This medicine puts you in an altered state. If you have no one to process with, to cry with because you have become the container for so much pain, then you will get into deep trouble. In Mexico, where the healers are supported by the community, as soon as the curandera is finished, a group of women will sprinkle holy water in a circle around her, and sprinkle specially prepared water on her neck, or massage her. They know that the curandera needs her energy to be replenished, and they honor that. When I first went to Mexico and observed how the healers were treated there, I felt so lonely. That's another reason why I knew that I needed apprentices, because I needed to create a viable support system for myself.

In the classes I created for my apprentices, we did in-depth work on many of the processes that we had studied at Ghost Ranch. We began by refining our techniques in conducting *pláticas*. I would ask for a volunteer, and one of my students who had something that she needed to talk about would agree to be the subject. One apprentice would be in charge of conducting the *plática*, while the others gathered round and listened. One of the most important things I taught was that this was not psychotherapy, but a listening from the heart. I actually had to do quite a bit of untraining of those who already had academic degrees in nursing or psychology. Sometimes the longest journey we make is the sixteen inches from our heads to our hearts. Periodically I would stop the *plática* and invite the whole class to discuss what was happening.

As my students progressed, I asked them to do *limpias* for their close friends and family. Practicing what they were learning was very important to their growth as healers, and I invited them to bring back their feedback and their feelings following such experiences. Because my apprentices were so insecure about what they were doing in the beginning, it was very helpful for them to begin by practicing on people who cared about them and had so much faith in them. Learning about *pláticas* created a stronger foundation for conducting more *limpias*. In that first year we also covered all the folk diseases, *susto, envídia, bilis, empacho,* and *mal ojo.* Because some of my students had jobs outside of the healing professions, they could not become full-time healers, so I tried to help them to find ways to incorporate what they were learning into their work. I had thought that we would get to soul retrievals, but there just wasn't time in that first year. We had to move at the pace of the group.

During this process, my apprentices were learning how to heal themselves, and we became a very close-knit community. All of their classes would take place in the "blue room," the place where I do all of my own healing with clients. Working there was very important for my students because it enabled them to experience the energy in that room and to be close to my altar. Soon they were calling our classes the Blue Room College.

In the first year, I didn't want to be the only one doing the teaching. I wanted my students to get as broad a perspective as possible, so I brought in many other teachers. I invited Dr. Oscar Hutterer, the president of the Mexican Academy of Traditional Medicine, to share his experiences of growing up around indigenous healers, his decision to abandon those beliefs when he went to medical school, and how he came full circle, returning to a healthy respect for curanderismo. He invited us to attend the Congress of Traditional Medicine where indigenous healers, herbalists, alternative health-care practitioners, and medical doctors all talk about their specialties. Since then, my students and I have attended the congress twice.

Dr. Eliseo Torres, author of two books on curanderismo and vice president of student affairs at the University of New Mexico, also came to speak with us. The writer of *Green Medicine: Traditional Mexican-American Herbal Remedies*, Dr. Torres is an expert on herbs. He brought many plants to my class, from both Mexico and the U.S., and discussed their uses. A curandera named Flordemayo, who practices Mayan indigenous healing and is an initiated Mayan priestess, came to talk to us about her medicine. She made it possible for us to attend a special ceremony at the village of her teacher Don Alejandro, the spiritual leader of the Quiché Maya in Guatemala. My sister Irma Martinez presented a class on the Mayan calendar and gave each student her Mayan name. Bernadette Vigil, a nagual shaman from the Eagle Knight lineage, assisted me in presenting my students with their medicine bags. I also brought in a woman named Pacal who is a descendant of Yaqui and Tarahumare Indians. Pacal took us all into the sweat lodge ceremony that she conducted.

Ehekateotl and his apprentice Tzenwaxolokuauhtli came to stay in my home for a week, and my apprentices and I helped them set up a clinic. Assisting Ehe and Tzen created a wonderful opportunity for my students to help with translations for patients who did not speak Spanish, and to observe these two Aztec healers in their work. This was also a great opportunity for them to learn lessons about community. My apprentices cooked meals, answered the phone to set up appointments, cleaned the house, and trafficked the tremendous numbers of people who came in for treatment. I was very proud of how my students pitched in.

When my students asked me to teach them for another year, I had to take some time off and think about it for a

while, but I finally agreed. This year we have been concen-
trating on soul retrievals. Slowly but surely, I have been loos-
ening my grip on my students, allowing them to do more and
more work on their own. I am also sending them referrals. If
someone calls me with a physical problem, I refer him to the
nurses in the group. If someone needs physical therapy, I refer him to the Rolfers or massage therapists in the group. This
year I am urging my students to become more independent,
to trust their intuition, and to start practicing curanderismo
more.

Going Back to the Root of the Medicine

One of the things that I made a requirement for the apprentices was that they go to Mexico so that they could see, feel,
and smell the root of where this medicine came from. I
wanted them to go to the *mercados,* the stores where I buy my
supplies, and to see stall after stall of medicinal herbs and
flowers. At the *mercado,* you can get remedies for any ailment
imaginable, and the people who sell the herbs are very experienced in their uses. I also wanted my apprentices to experience how accessible curanderismo is in Mexico. I wanted
them to see the amulets, the special soaps that attract lovers
and those that make them go away, the bath powders for
good luck, the many types of sacred candles for sale that have
been blessed by curanderas. I showed them how to shop for
the specially prepared waters and the freshly harvested copal
that I use in my ceremonies. They were like kids in a candy
store, shopping and shopping.

I took my students to my teacher Ehekateotl's *kalpulli*

(school). There we were received by all of his students and apprentices, who had prepared a feast of incredibly delicious food. We ate tamales prepared in the Yucatán style, wrapped in banana leaves, and enjoyed many other traditional dishes. The comadres and compadres welcomed us with a beautiful blessing and ceremony in front of the altar, and a talking circle in which they said many wonderful and welcoming things to us.

One of the most amazing parts of the experience was getting permission to do a sweat lodge at a place called Xochimilco, which is a place of floating gardens and islands. The government had made it into a tourist spot filled with colorful boats and mariachi bands, but recently the Aztecs have been granted permission to have their traditional sweat lodges on some of the sacred islands. We loaded all the supplies we would need for a sweat lodge ceremony onto two of the beautifully painted long gondolas that are for rent, and floated for an hour through the narrow canals while the Aztec healers played flutes and drums and sang enchanting songs. Once we had arrived, we transported all of our wood, water, and supplies to the site, and then worked for hours covering the sweat lodge with tall grasses that we harvested ourselves. Each stone was held up and blessed before it was placed in the fire pit. Some of the elder men and women told us that there had not been a *temazcal* (sweat lodge) ceremony on that location for three hundred and fifty years. As the special instrument that made the sound of the eagle's cry whistled and the flutes played, we all chanted sacred words in Nahuatl. It felt as if the spirits from three centuries ago were with us.

I felt that it was extremely important for my students to

visit the four ancient power places of the Aztecs in Mexico City. It's one thing to do the directions in ceremony, but these are the places where the energy originated, and I wanted them to stand at the source. For thousands of years, the Aztec peoples had done ceremony at these sacred sites, and they had continued to do so, even after the Spaniards conquered the ancient Aztec city of Tenochtitlán, the old name for what today we call Mexico City. What many people do not realize is that, unlike many indigenous people faced with the violence of the conqueror, the Aztecs did not leave. They stayed in their sacred city, and continued to honor and do ceremony at the power places of the four directions. As so often happens, the Spaniards, in their effort to stamp out the old religion, built their own churches on top of these sites, but even this did not stop the Aztecs from honoring these places with their ceremonies and dances.

I had planned our trip so that we could be in Mexico City on December 12, the feast day of the Virgin of Guadalupe. We were very honored and blessed to be invited by a group of Aztecs to a pilgrimage and an all-night vigil at the basilica. The dark-skinned Virgin of Guadalupe is a very important figure to both Mexicans and Americans. As the story goes, she appeared to an indigenous man and told him that she wanted a church in her honor to be built at the base of the hill. When the Indian tried to tell the priest about his vision, no one would believe him. To help him to prove his story, the Virgin filled his cloak with beautiful fragrant roses in the dead of winter. When the priest saw the miracle of the roses, he believed, and he erected the church. The Virgin of Guadalupe is the most beloved of all saints in Mexico, and also, in the eyes of many curanderas, their patron saint. In 1754, she was declared Patroness and Protectress of New Spain. Today, the Basilica of Guadalupe is situated at the foot of Tepeyac Hill, in Mexico City, in the same place where the shrine to the Aztec goddess of earth and corn, Tonatzin, stood.

Being present at the feast day of the Virgin of Guadalupe was a very moving experience for me and my students. There were thousands and thousands of people there. Many had walked all the way on their knees, hundreds of miles, to ask for a miracle. It is an awesome sight to see the humility and acts of faith of these people who have come from all over the world to make this pilgrimage. Instead of walking, some had even rolled their bodies sideways along the ground for the last few miles. The sight moved us to tears, and many of my students told me afterward that it had spiritually strengthened them to see such acts of faith, and to see the thousands of people gathered in one place to honor the Virgin.

The feast day of the Virgin really starts on the evening of December 11 when many circles of Aztec tribes celebrate all-night vigils with drumming and chanting. The next day the Aztec dancers do ceremony and dance all day. It's quite a beautiful experience to see all of the colored sacred clothes and the headdresses covered with long feathers. Because I had danced at this basilica with Andres Segura back in the eighties, watching these dances brought back incredible memories. All of these experiences had a profound impact on my students, moving them to an incredible place, and teaching them the lesson that you can't separate the medicine from its cultural roots.

Traveling to the Holy Mountain: Humor and Adversity

One of the most important events on our trip was the journey we took to one of the holy mountains of the Aztecs. My teacher Ehekateotl had arranged for a welcoming lunch for us at the restaurant of a friend named Antonio, a curandero who healed through nutrition. Antonio would be cooking our meals for us throughout the trip. At the restaurant, we were also going to meet Flor Silvestre, one of Ehe's apprentices, who, along with Antonio, was going to be our guide on the trip.

The plan was that, after lunch, we would get on a bus together and go to a sacred site in a town called Chalma at the foot of the mountain, about two hours south of Mexico City. After a ceremony at Chalma, Antonio and Flor were going to guide us to a sun-dance ground at the top of the mountain. This was a very special place built by a North Native American who had introduced the sun dance to the Aztecs and gifted them with a sun-dance ground on top of this special mountain. We were to meet with the keeper of the mountain, Tata Faustino, an elder who had prepared supper and a sweat lodge for us.

Our schedule was tight because two days later, I was scheduled to present a paper at the national conference of the Academia Mexicana de Medicina Tradicional. Not only that but my students and I were to be honored with a ceremony during which we would receive our Nahuatl names following the conference.

I had entrusted the agenda for our week to one of my apprentices, Soledad. Meanwhile, Ehe had given our bus driver explicit instructions about the name of the restaurant and how to get there. Antonio's restaurant was in the center of Mexico City, a huge metropolis many consider even larger and more complex to navigate in than New York City. The whole time the bus driver kept shaking his head, "Oh, *sí, señor,* I know exactly where this restaurant is." Since he was from Mexico City, I didn't worry. I figured he knew what he was talking about.

We were all staying at a bed-and-breakfast in the middle of Mexico City where every morning we would do our talking circle and then get ready for our next adventure. That morning the bus driver picked us up, and what began as a pleasant journey became a nightmare. It became obvious that we were driving in circles around Mexico City. I finally asked the driver if he knew where he was taking us, and he said, "I think the name of the restaurant is Fernandos." I said, "But you were so sure when Ehe was giving you instructions." He said, "Don't worry, we'll find it."

We circled around for an hour or so, and it became very clear that he had no idea where this restaurant was. I instructed him to stop and ask for directions, but no one had heard of Fernandos. Finally I came up with a "spiritual plan." We would find the restaurant by doing the *cruz*, the cross of the four directions. We all piled out of the bus and I announced, "One of the reasons we are in Mexico is to honor the power places at the four directions. So some of you go in a radius of several blocks in the south and ask for directions to Fernandos restaurant." I gave the other comadres the same instructions for each point of the compass. We planned to meet back at the bus at a prearranged time. I was sure that the ancestors would guide us magically to Fernandos.

The bus driver, Roberto, looked at us as if we were crazy, lit a cigarette, and hunkered down to wait. At this point, I was very angry with him and did not want to talk to him anyway. About half an hour later, we all rendezvoused back at the bus. Unfortunately, nobody had found Fernandos restaurant. We couldn't call and ask Ehe for help because he and the whole tribe had already left for the town of Oaxtepec, Morelos, where the academy's conference was being held, and he was going to present a paper.

By this time, we were getting hungry and upset. My students saw my agitation and began to offer advice, which was the last thing I wanted to hear at this point. "Maybe this just wasn't supposed to be, comadre. Maybe we should give up and go back to the bed-and-breakfast." I was not willing to give up yet, and I told my students to leave me alone. I have always been very sensitive and I could *sense* Antonio and Flor waiting and worrying about us. I could feel their great concern about the responsibility they had to take us to all these places, and imagined them sitting there at the restaurant, wringing their hands, surrounded by piles of food.

We finally went to a nearby park and bought some snacks and sodas. I sat down by myself and prayed to Spirit for direction. I knew my students felt badly for me, and wanted to help, but I also knew that I had to figure out what to do. I clearly saw the impossibility of our ever finding the restaurant. There we were in the heart of Mexico City with 19 million people around us and three restaurants on every block. I sensed the futility of even trying to find Fernandos. I finally told the bus driver to take us to the power place of the west.

I thought that maybe, by some act of God, we would find Flor and Antonio there. I also knew where Chalma was. I figured that if we could just get that far, I could somehow figure out how to get us to the top of the mountain. I did not want to disappoint Tata Faustino, the elder who was also waiting for us. I thought that at least that way we could meet up with *one* of our guides. Somehow, by some miracle, maybe the other two would be there waiting for us.

When we got back onto the bus, I asked Soledad to hand me the schedule. She looked at me with chagrin, and said, "*Maestra,* I've lost it." I gave her a withering look. Nothing was going right that day.

We did manage to reach the power place of the west, and did a very incredible ceremony there. One of the things my students noticed was that there was no symbol of Aztec spirituality in that place. There was a tremendous cathedral that towered above that little town like an archangel, but not one thing that indicated that this spot was sacred to the Aztecs, except for a small circle of Aztec dancers who were also doing a ceremony there.

By this time, it was getting dark, but I was still determined to go to Chalma. The bus driver looked at me anxiously and reminded me that it was a two-hour drive and that there were no motels. Nevertheless, I was determined to go. I saw a telephone booth with a telephone book, so I called our bed-and-breakfast to try one last time to see if there had been any messages left for us by Flor and Antonio. There were none.

By this time, I was in tears, thinking about all of those people who were worried about us. At this point, some of my students came out of the bus and gently and lovingly persuaded me to surrender. They said, "Please, *maestra,* you're tired, we're tired. Let's go back to the hotel and see what happens tomorrow." At that point, I realized that they were my teachers. I really did have to give up my own will and surrender.

The next morning after breakfast, we were finishing our morning ceremony in the living room of Casa Gonzales. Just then, the French doors opened and a beautiful, dark-skinned, long-haired woman came in wearing a huipile. She looked confused, as if she had *susto.* Then she saw the nineteen women in the circle and smelled the copal. She called out, "Elena? Elena?" I came out of the circle and took her in my arms. She burst out crying. "Oh, we were so worried about you. We waited for hours and hours yesterday. It took me so long to find you. I knew your hotel was called Casa Gonzales, but I couldn't find it in the phone book. I finally walked up and down the street, looking for it, until someone told me where it was."

This was a great lesson for my students. They could see how these people had been suffering, how they had been looking for us for twenty-four hours, not giving up their responsibility to take care of us. There was great learning on all sides. Flor called Antonio and told him to pack up all the food. We went to the restaurant, picked him up, and all headed for Chalma.

It was difficult for some of the women to get up that mountain because of the altitude, the long hard climb, some physical difficulties that some of the comadres had, and the fact that we were carrying all that food. But we helped each other make it. By the time we reached the top, however, it was dark. Tata Faustino had other obligations, so he could not meet us, but he had asked two of his helpers to be there waiting for us.

We cooked our food by moonlight and prepared our bedding up in the loft in a barn. The mountain got very cold, and we didn't have enough sleeping bags, so we ended up not sleeping all night. This was a difficult experience for many of my students, but they learned from it. Many of them came up to me afterward and said, "*Maestra,* now we understand a little bit of what you have gone through all these years. We understand all the nights you suffered, all of the things you have done over the years to be able to learn and to offer us this medicine." It was a beautiful experience in which many tears were shared.

It took us a long time to get down from that mountain, and of course there was no place or time for bathing, but we all felt united as we made the descent. Of course, I still had to present my paper, and it was a two-hour drive to Oaxtepec. We were very late and, at this point, the whole congress was worried about us. By the time we arrived, Dr. Hutterer was at the point of agitation, "Where were you?!" he yelled. He had rearranged the schedule so that I would present my paper right before lunch, but it was later than that now. Everyone in the audience was falling asleep and lethargic. I woke them all up, however, and made them laugh with my presentation on *envídia.*

Afterward, we all went to the town of Cocoyoc, a place of gardens and hot springs where Aztec royalty used to go for relaxation. Ehe had arranged an exquisite ceremony for us to receive our Nahuatl names. Accompanied by Aztec dancers, drums, and flutes, we marched in procession into an incredibly beautiful location. Everyone was dressed in brilliant colors in their ceremonial clothing and feathered headdresses.

Because I had wanted to look semiprofessional for the presentation at the Congress, I had taken off my stinky panties on the bus and put pantyhose on under my long tight skirt. While we were in the circle, Ehe gestured to me to take off my pantyhose so that I would be barefoot with my feet touching the earth. Needless to say, I was extremely worried about how I was going to manage this feat of gracefully taking off my pantyhose without mooning everyone present, but I managed somehow. Some things are non-negotiable, and having pantyhose between my feet and Mother Earth was one of them.

The ceremony was exquisitely beautiful. Ehe gave each of us our Nahuatl names, and then struck our hands and feet with a special decorated staff, repeating our names several times to plant them in our bodies. I had already received the first part of my Nahuatl name, Xochitl, which means "flower." This name was derived from the date of my birth. On this day, Ehe gave me the rest of my name, Xochitl-wetzkapahtli (Flower That Attracts and Brings Medicine Through Laughter). During the time that we had known each other, he had been observing my soul, and he had seen what the Aztecs call my "true face and heart." The name he had chosen for me reflected that. One of the things that he told me was that this name represented a lot of responsibility for me. He cautioned me that if I did not respect my responsibilities, the community could also take my name away from me. He gave each of us a medicine necklace with the symbol of our names on it. My students were touched and transformed that someone would go to such trouble for them, setting up such an amazing ceremony.

What a lesson this day was, and how appropriate that my name would include the concept of laughter. I had had to go through all the crazy experiences of the past two days just to learn not only that I needed to make people laugh, but that I also had to learn to laugh at myself. This naming ceremony was also a kind of soul retrieval for me. As he pounded my name into my hands and feet, all of my names flashed through my mind, Ada, Elenita, Helen, Elena. We get our first names from the Aztec calendar, but only a teacher can give us our whole name.

It was a week of incredible experiences, and it seemed as if my comadres and I had spent a lifetime there. For many of us, it was hard coming back to the day-to-day world in the U.S. after seeing so much magic and sharing in so many blessings with such a kind and loving community of people.

The Eagle's Gift

Recently my students and I had one more incredible experience together atop a sacred mountain outside of Chichicastenango called Pascual Abaj, one of the most sacred sites in Guatemala. For several months, Dr. Hutterer and his wife, Rachel, had been caring for an eagle that had been injured. It had molted some feathers and Rachel had asked me if my students were ready to receive their eagle feathers. I had said no at the time, but now, as we prepared to make our trip to Guatemala, I told Rachel that the time had come for me to present my apprentices with their feathers. Eagle feathers are a very special tool for the healer because they are considered sacred. An eagle feather is given to a healer by another healer or elder when a readiness is observed. It is a great honor to be given an eagle feather. My students had just finished the first year of their apprenticeship, and now they were ready. What was also very meaningful to me was that the eagle the feathers had come from had completely healed and had finally flown away.

Ehe asked a Lakota medicine man and a medicine man from Ecuador to assist him in the ceremony. Many participants from the Congress of Traditional Medicine, which was held in Quetzaltenango that year, went up the mountain with us. At the time, my students had no idea that they were going to receive an eagle feather. All they knew was that we planned to do some kind of ceremony honoring them. I found out later that some of them had even been talking among themselves, feeling self-conscious, saying, "I don't know why they are doing a special ceremony for us. We don't need a ceremony." Hearing this, my coauthor, Joy Parker, who was with us on this trip, was dying inside, thinking, "My God, don't you know that you are all going to be honored with your first eagle feathers?" but she didn't say a word to them about it.

At the top of the mountain, we formed two circles, an outer circle where my apprentices and I stood, and an inner circle of elders and medicine people. One by one, Ehe called out the Nahuatl names of apprentices. I led them, one at a time, into the inner circle where Ehe spoke some personal words to them. Then the medicine people all blessed the eagle feathers and Ehe lovingly handed them to each student.

Finally there was one extra feather left. Ehe called me over and handed it to me, saying, "You have just given birth to your first generation. This is a big responsibility. You will be responsible for what they say and what they do with this medicine for the rest of your life." I felt overwhelmed with gratitude and also with a knowledge of the immensity of what I had undertaken, to pass on what I had learned to a new generation of curanderas.

When I first set out to teach, I had thought it would be so easy. As a person born in the spring, which is the season of the east, I am always filled with optimism and grand ideas. Mystery has always beckoned to me, and I have always gone to the unknown for unknown reasons. In my early years teaching at Ghost Ranch, and with my first batch of apprentices, I made a lot of mistakes. I will continue with the students that I have now for as long as they need me, but I don't know if I will even take on a new group of students. That is one of the mysteries of my future. I feel, however, that I have finally learned some wisdom that will keep me from making some of the same mistakes, such as giving people sacred tools before they are ready for them. No doubt, however, I will make new ones because we are all always in a process of learning.

Being presented with an eagle feather on that mountaintop in Guatemala was like coming full circle. I remembered how I had prayed for an eagle feather for years, back in my early days when I practiced the medicine and went back and forth to Mexico to study. The feather that Ehe gave to me was the fifth I had received from medicine people. I knew that, symbolically, I had traveled the full hoop, had gone to all of the four directions and arrived at the fifth direction, the center.

Chapter Seven

The Gods That Refused to Die
The Future of the Medicine of the People

In the year 1521, after the Spaniards had invaded Mexico and destroyed the ancient capital of Tenochtitlán, the Aztec people saw that a time of darkness was coming. In a famous proclamation that has been preserved for nearly five hundred years, Cuauhtémoc, the last ruler of the Aztec Empire, put forth a desperate plan to preserve what he could of his people's spiritual and cultural beliefs. He told them to destroy their ballcourts, their places of learning, their sacred temples, and their power places and to take everything that they considered a treasure, everything that was precious and important to them, and place it deep within their hearts. Mothers and fathers were instructed to preserve their knowledge secretly within their homes and to teach their children the spiritual, philosophical, and medicinal ways of the people. In this way, even though their "sun was now in darkness," the knowledge that the Aztec civilization had gathered over the long years of their civilization could be protected until the time when their prophecies foretold that their sun would rise again.

The coming of the Conquistadores was a time of great anguish, destruction, and soul loss for the Aztecs. There is a story about the *tlamatinime,* the Aztec wise men, that illustrates how devastating it is to rob people of their culture and their spiritual beliefs. After all of their power places and sacred sites had been destroyed and the Spaniards had told them that the Christian God was the only one that they could worship, the *tlamatinime* were called to appear before Hernán Cortés and the legendary Twelve Friars. "If, as you say, our gods are dead," they said, "it is better that you allow us to die too." But the "gods,"—the energy forces that the Aztecs honored—refused to die, as did the medicine and the spirituality of the people. I myself and the many others alive in the world today who honor the old ways are living proof that much has survived.

In 1992, the five-hundredth year following Columbus's discovery of America, I was witness to how strongly the Aztecs had resisted those forces that had tried to annihilate their culture. During the week of October 12, indigenous people from all over the world gathered together in Mexico City to protest the honor being done to Columbus for his acts of violence and genocide. Most of all, they were protesting the fact that, historically, it was not well recognized that people with rich cultures and highly developed medicinal systems were already living in the New World long before the Europeans had arrived. This gathering represented a true pilgrimage. Groups of indigenous people from all over the world were present, and many from North, South, and Central America had made the long journey on foot. One group of Indians from Alaska had walked for an entire year to get there.

I was there with a group from New Mexico. On our first evening together, many of us did ceremony in Teotihuacán, the ancient city that the Aztecs had named, "the place where men became gods." At one time, Teotihuacán was one of the most influential religious and political sites in all of Meso-America. It was also the site of one of the Spaniards' greatest military defeats, the Noche Triste (Sad Night). Dressed in colorful clothing, playing musical instruments, dancing and doing ceremony, people from many different cultures poured into this awesome city surrounded by three huge structures, the Pyramid of the Sun, the Pyramid of the Moon, and the Pyramid of Quetzalcoatl.

The next day, we all returned to the heart of Mexico City, the Zócalo, also known as the Plaza de la Constitución, one of the largest plazas in the world. The Zócalo is special to the Aztecs because so much of their history lies buried beneath it. Spaniards began to lay out this square immediately after the conquest of Tenochtitlán, the ancient Aztec name for Mexico City. Half of this plaza was built over the southern part of the demolished Aztec temple precinct, the Teocalli. In the northern part of this plaza stands the building that is known simply as "the cathedral," one of the largest churches in the Western Hemisphere. This imposing and beautiful structure, built in

1563, is crowned with two high steeples. Built over the site of another ancient temple that the Spaniards demolished, the cathedral is sacred ground to the Aztecs.

On this day, many beautiful ceremonies with dancing and singing were being celebrated in front of this building. As the Zócalo filled with the smell of copal and hundreds of people drummed, one Aztec warrior began to climb up the outside of the cathedral. Hundreds of thousands of people watched and cheered him on, their faces uplifted. When he got up to the top of the highest steeple, he leaned out and let out a yell, "We did not die!" I will never forget that moment as long as I live.

If you listen to the Incas or the Mayas, and all of the indigenous people on the continents of North and South America, you will hear the same story. Although the Europeans tried to destroy their way of life, it refused to die. If the gods refused to die, the culture refused to die, and the medicine refused to die, then there still must be a purpose for it. I don't believe it is an accident that a Chicana born and raised in the U.S. with a master's degree in nursing is still practicing the medicine that was passed down from generation to generation, the medicine of my ancestors.

The time has come when more and more indigenous healers are beginning to share their medicine. African medicine man Malidoma Somé was told by his elders to share some of their knowledge in the workshops that he gives around the world and in his books *Of Water and the Spirit* and *The Healing Wisdom of Africa*. Shaman Martín Prechtel was told by his Tzutujil Mayan teacher to return to the "land of the dead," the United States, to share the knowledge of ceremony and healing that he had been given. He has also shared his story in *Secrets of the Talking Jaguar*. We can all think of many, many other indigenous men and women who, in recent times, have been instructed by their elders to teach their medicine in books, gatherings, ceremonies, and workshops.

In the speech that he made before the 1997 Congress of Traditional Medicine, my teacher Ehekateotl referred back to the words of the last Aztec ruler, telling us that his people believed that the time of cultural rebirth was at hand. The time of sharing with the children of the conqueror that Cuauhtémoc had prophesied was now upon us.

"The Aztecs did not share their 'greatest medicine' with the Spaniards because it became very evident that the Spaniards would misunderstand our spiritual beliefs," Ehekateotl told the 1997 Congress of Traditional Medicine. "Our medicine was our great treasure and we have guarded it carefully because we knew it would be destroyed otherwise. In the year 1521, Cuauhtémoc, the last ruler of the Aztec Empire and grand bearer of the oral tradition, urged that the writings and wisdom of the ancient Mexihka be preserved in the heart of the family descendants of the Aztecs. The people accepted this order and the responsibility of guarding and maintaining this knowledge intact. These teachings were transmitted from father to son, and from mother to daughter. This tradition was guarded jealously for 468 years, which was the period of transformation. But now, we initiate the new period of development and growth in which we can share this knowledge. . . .

Another time, Ehe related a story about his father. "My father was born in the city of Mexico, as was all my family, for more than six hundred years. He was a person of great and profound consciousness about our tradition. For fifty-two years, he was responsible for a tradition called Mexihko Tlaltonaltikeh, which means 'The one who captures the shadow in Mexico.' For that reason, during all that time, he could not travel outside the Mexico City area. His obligation did not permit it. He practiced the medicine in a form that was marvelous because he was a man with integrity, and he provided a service to his community. He educated people in the development of the science of astronomy and in the system of using our calendar, and in agriculture and commerce. He lived during an epoch that was the last of the occultation [the darkening of the sun]. He could not use his authentic name, he could not freely wear his traditional clothes, but had to wear a suit and a tie. The tradition was concealed [from the outside world] for more than 468 years, and my father died seven years before we could disclose it. The ancestors had already determined that this time would come in 1989."

For me, the return of the medicine of the Aztecs, and the reemergence of folk medicine into the modern world, is no small matter. As a curandera who is constantly striving to learn from other cultures, especially from my Mexican and indigenous roots, the rebirth of folk medicine is something that touches me, my students, my clients, and my community every day of my life.

The Man with the Knife

Recently Western culture's need for the wisdom of folk healers and the skills of the practitioners of alternative medicine affected me in a very dramatic and personal way. On April 24, 1998, I had surgery to remove a fatty tumor the size of a golf ball from the right side of my neck. It had been growing steadily larger for over a year. An ear, nose, and throat specialist whom I went to recommended that it be excised. I agreed because the tumor was starting to give me some sharp shooting pains. The doctor told me that it was a very simple surgery that would require a local anesthesia and take forty minutes. That was all he had to say about the procedure.

During the surgery, I realized that the resident, not the specialist, was doing the actual surgery, but I was too numb and drugged to protest. I do remember hearing the doctor say, "This tumor is much bigger than I thought." I went home about two hours later and, by ten o'clock that night, started to worry because the anesthesia had not worn off. I felt numbness all over my right ear, the right side of my jaw, and the side and back of my neck. At midnight I phoned the surgeon on call. He bluntly said, "The anesthesia wore off hours ago. They must have cut a nerve. The feeling in your face and neck might or might not come back."

I had a hard time sleeping that night, wondering what it would be like to not have sensation on that side of my face and neck for the rest of my life. Would I have to teach my grandchildren to kiss me only on the left side of my face and neck, tell my lover that his caresses on that side would not reach my heart? Every time I turned to my right side, which is my favorite sleeping position, I felt as if a foreign object was poking in my face. This sensation would startle me until I realized that this was my own ear. My brain was telling me that my ear was a foreign object.

Six days later I went back to the doctor's office to have my stitches removed. When the doctor breezed in and asked me how I was doing, I burst out crying, saying, "I can't feel that side of my face. Did you cut the nerve? Is this condition permanent?"

The doctor immediately went on the defensive. He said, "I can't really predict what is going to happen. I don't know if the numbness is permanent or temporary. It takes a long time for nerves to come back. The nerve may not come back for months, or ever. If you don't have any feeling in a year and a half, then I will begin to worry." This statement filled me with incredible sadness. I thought, "Is it going to take this doctor a year and a half to care about what his knife did to me?" I also asked myself, "Is this the kind of medicine that we want for ourselves, for our families, for our old people and our children? Is this the best that we can do?"

Fortunately I know medicines greater than this, and I knew where to look for the help that I really needed. I went to my Mexican acupuncturist, Olivario Pijoan, and he was loving and attentive to me. He took out an anatomy book, sat down next to me, and showed me the possible neural pathways that might have been injured or destroyed. He also told me that, in the past, he has successfully repaired some of the damage that medical doctors have done. Most important, he assured me that, working together, we would be able to get the feeling back in my face. After his treatment, I received a loving massage from the massage therapist in his office.

One of the most healing experiences that I had was receiving the *yerba-buena* words of my dear friend Kaiya that she sent to me via E-mail. *Yerba buena* is a term that Chicanos use to refer to any kind of medicine that is lovingly administered by a grandmother, mother, or healer. People have written me beautiful words before in letters and E-mails, but this was the first time I'd ever been woken up so powerfully to the realization that I had the power within myself to be medicine, to create my own healing. Kaiya's loving, healing, medicine

words guided me to go within and do a soul retrieval, to call
back all the parts of myself that had gone into hiding during
this terrible experience. I will share some of her remarkable
letter with you here:

"Elena, I am so glad that you got acupuncture and massage
for your face and neck. But I am again asking you to take the
words of the physician that took you to the knife and put
them in a compost pile with many other healing experiences.
One of the things that I think your nursing education and experience did was to make you much too susceptible to M.D.
authority. You repeat his words 'months or ever' as if they
were truths. . . . Simply put, [he and his intern] don't know
exactly what they did and they don't know exactly how to fix
it, or even if it will fix itself.

"This is where your selective listening comes in. The body
seeks the truth. The body, like water going through a dry
rocky stream, seeks to unite itself with the damaged parts.
Your role inside the body is to listen to this water and try to
remove the boulders of fear and the rocks of M.D. negativity
and impersonalization by relaxing the energetic patterns so
that the nerves can reconnect the fibers of their tapestry. The
more stress and anxiety [you feel,] the more difficult will be
the natural energetic flow.

"My dear sister, become the wind and breathe away the
stress into dust whirls in the desert. Come to the ocean that
once caressed the desert floor. Let the water lead you through
the sweat, herbal baths, trips to the healing hot springs. Kiss
the fire with the sweet scents of copal, sage, cedar and whatever calls you to the *limpia*, carrying the signals of your pain,
fear, and anxiety on the clouds of smoke to signal the ancestors of your need for their support. And lie on the earth, my

Elena. Cover yourself with mud, feel the power of the Mother's fibers under your feet in the plants you surround yourself with. Feel her as the Spiderwoman re-creating the necessary web that has only been damaged by a small intrusion. Perhaps this is a draining time, necessary to release the psychic debris associated with your tumor creation. Let it become stardust, Elena. Let your authentic self reconnect to your smile, not to your paralysis, the unfeeling protection of the invaded self. You are now creating who you are, the artist at work.

"Audre Lorde in *The Cancer Journals* talks about this paralyzing fear. 'For we have been socialized to respect fear more than our own needs for language and definition, and while we wait in silence for that final luxury of fearlessness the weight of that silence will choke us.'

"Sing it out. Dance it out, *mi compañera, mi hermana curandera.* We are the ones we have been waiting for. Release your voice, move your stiff neck with the bending of the willow as it seeks the water of life. Know that the circle never ends and that we are all one. *En paz, salud y amor, siempre,* Kaiya."

Reading this letter, which arrived with such synchronicity during the writing of the final chapter of this book, I realized that perhaps the time had come for me to move even further away from Western medicine. Looking back, I realized that I needed to undo some of my nursing training, to lose some of the unqualified respect that I was taught in the presence of the all-powerful Western doctor. I realized that perhaps I had submitted to the knife too quickly. Perhaps I should have tried alternative therapies first, healers who would have helped me to shrink the tumor, or at least to find out the reasons why my body is growing these lipomas. When I asked the medical doctor why I was producing tumors, he told me that he had no idea. This was the third tumor they have found in my body, and the last two were discovered within the space of a year.

Western medicine is capable of doing many helpful things. There are many technological advances that are mind-boggling in their ability to heal things we could never heal before. There are many doctors who *are* loving and *do* take time to be with their patients. I am not saying that we should throw all of this way. I am only saying that the time has come when we need to take a long, hard look at the modern medical system that we have created, acknowledge its strengths and weaknesses, and then see what our alternatives are. Most important, we need to look long and hard at how quickly we are willing, as I was, to give away our power to doctors without really exploring these alternatives.

How Modern Medicine Perceives Alternative Medicine

It is ironic that while I, as a curandera, am willing to use Western medicine as a complement to my own, Western medicine sees alternative and folk medicine as scientifically unproven or unorthodox. Although alternative therapies have been practiced effectively for hundreds of years and widely utilized in the treatment and diagnosis of diseases, the scientifically oriented medical establishment has been skeptical about them, and sometimes even strongly opposed to their use. Medical doctors even question the value of herbs such as echinacea and St. John's wort, the effectiveness of which has now been conclusively proven in scientific trials.

Lately the trend away from folk and alternative medicine has been reversing itself somewhat. In 1993, the U.S. National Institutes of Health established the Office of Alternative Medicine to examine the merits of medicines such as curanderismo, chiropractic, homeopathy, acupuncture, herbal medicine, meditation, biofeedback, massage therapy, and much more. Nevertheless, the regulation of herbs that we have used for centuries to heal ourselves is now being controlled by the government. The American Medical Association has tremendous power over our health care, and the lay person has to abide by the rules and regulations set forth by this system. Managed health care companies determine how long your doctor visit will be, what tests you will have, how long your hospital stay will be, and if you can be referred to another doctor. Pregnant women are being discharged twenty-four hours after delivery. For some women and their newborn children, this has had negative repercussions. It is almost impossible to find an insurance company that will pay for care from an alternative healer.

In this book I have raised the question of how conventional medicine and curanderismo can work together. The truth is, this complementary partnership can exist only if the modern doctor is able to have a genuine attitude of respect toward folk healing, and a genuine interest in its healing modalities. Most physicians do not want to incorporate into their course of treatment a health system that cannot be defined by a linear, scientific approach. While I refer many of my clients to medical doctors, and/or make myself available to work with them in the context of a team, I rarely hear from a doctor who is interested in working with me for the health of a patient.

A major barrier to the cooperation of doctors and folk/alternative healers is the modern doctor's belief that diseases are caused by specific versus nonspecific (such as emotional and soul) factors. For example, if you ask a modern doctor what causes stomach ulcers, he will say "a bacteriological infection," and will try to cure it with antibiotics. According to many doctors, a holistic approach that includes such general things as diet, emotions, spirit, and work on the personality is a waste of time and money, and will only slow down the quick cure promised by the fast-acting antibiotics. How can we argue with such logic? Of course, there are patients who do not want holistic care. They just want the antibiotic for their ulcer, and their wishes should be respected. They are fortunate to have a medical system that supports their desires. Quick cure, case closed.

The Course of Treatment in a Modern HMO

If we look at the broader picture of how ulcers are dealt with in the modern medical system, we see a much less efficient and effective process at work. First of all, under modern HMOs, most of us would have to wait two months to see our family physician. Since HMOs are in the business of saving money, before any expensive diagnostic tests could be run, the doctor would probably initially prescribe an acid-reducing drug. While waiting to see if the antacid is going to help his condition, the patient feels lousy and his energy is low. He no longer enjoys the pleasure of eating. His sleep is poor, and he is fighting with his wife because he feels bad, is cranky, and doesn't want to make love as often as he used to.

Two months later, still ill with severe stomach pains, he goes back to his doctor, who orders X-rays, an upper GI series, and a barium enema. The doctor diagnoses an ulcer, but refers the patient to a gastroenterology specialist for management of the disease. The patient waits two more months to see the specialist. In the meantime, his illness has taken a toll on his personal life and his work. If the patient has a negative reaction to the antibiotics that the gastroenterologist prescribes, he will be given a second medicine to counter the side-effects. If the patient is a woman, she might get a vaginal infection from the medication, and will need to be given a cream or a vaginal suppository to treat that complication. If the first prescription does not kill the bacteria and heal the ulcer, then another antibiotic will be prescribed.

The emotions or soul loss that result from having a bleeding ulcer, or the stress or emotional problems that might have caused it in the first place, will not even be considered in the treatment—unless the patient complains of depression, in which case the doctor will be happy to describe an antidepressant. If the antidepressant interferes with the patient's sex life, or makes him want to sleep all day, then there is another drug that can be taken in tandem with the antidepressant that will lessen those new side-effects. And so it goes.

There is an old joke that says much about where we have arrived with our current medical system. St. Peter is standing at the gates of heaven when three doctors approach. He asks the first doctor, "What have you done to get into heaven?"

The doctor replies, "I am a heart doctor and I have saved hundreds of lives."

St. Peter replies, "That's just great. You can enter heaven."

The next doctor says, "I have delivered thousands of healthy babies."

Saint Peter says, "Wonderful, you can come into heaven, too."

Finally the last doctor approaches and St. Peter asks, "And what have you done to get into heaven?"

That doctor replies, "I worked for a managed health-care company and saved them millions of dollars."

St. Peter replies, "Come on in. You get three days."

Collaborating with Sacred Medicine

During my years of speaking and traveling throughout Mexico and the U.S., I have come across some medical doctors with an extraordinary vision of how we can combine the best of both modern and ancient medicine. One outstanding example of this type of individual is Dr. Oscar Hutterer Ariza, a medical doctor of twenty-eight years who specializes in dermatology and psychiatry. Dr. Hutterer is a professor of medicine at the University of Mexico City where he teaches psychology and a course on the history and philosophy of medicine from the time of Hippocrates to the modern day.

Born in 1941 in Mexico City, the child of a German father and a mother from Veracruz, Mexico, Dr. Hutterer has lived in indigenous communities for much of his life. He was attracted to medicine at a very young age because he wanted to be useful. His lifelong interest in folk medicine began in childhood when his mother, who knew many of the remedies of homeopathy, often used the services of curanderos. He received *limpias* with the herb *pirul*, and was also treated by spiritualists.

When he attended the university, however, he was brainwashed into believing that folk medicine was superstition. "I was trained as a doctor to be abusive to patients who believed in popular medicine (curanderismo). I was taught that this medicine was for ignorant people and that, as doctors, we needed to destroy these practices. When I talked to patients who believed their child had *mal ojo,* I would correct them. 'Do not be a *burro,*' I would say. I was the *burro.* I was the ignorant one. But, even though I was educated to think this way, I was always interested in indigenous medicine."

As time went on, Dr. Hutterer began to rediscover the value of the medicine of his childhood and his pueblo. "My university training had been limited, focusing mainly on pharmacology. This kind of education impedes an equal relationship with patients. It does not permit physicians to recognize illness from the community's viewpoint, much less show them how to cure it. Doctors impose a therapeutic system upon people that is foreign to their culture. Our care is fragmented. This is why our patients do not get well. I realized very early in my career that I had not been trained to care for the illness of my pueblo. I had been educated to enrich the institutions that live from the pain of people, i.e., laboratories, pharmaceutical companies, hospitals, etc.

"In 1978 I founded the Academia Mexicana de Medicina Tradicional with a group of physicians and others who were dissatisfied with Western medicine. We all wanted to serve the pueblos better. Some of my critics laughed and told me that I was walking backward. But I knew better. When I was in medical school I attended my first delivery and noticed how painful it was for the mother. She was lying down and working against gravity. I saw women with torn uteruses, vaginal tears, and many complications. I remembered the pictures I had seen of indigenous women giving birth and realized that they had a superior method of delivery. I started to notice that I would cure my patients of one disease and give her another, many from the side-effects of the medication I prescribed. I observed curanderos treating illness and noticed that the *limpias*, herbs, and homeopathy caused minimal complications and secondary illnesses. I realized that my education was limited and that I had to learn other methods of healing. I started to integrate curanderismo with Western medicine."

There came a time when Dr. Hutterer wanted to gather together with other practitioners of traditional medicine, so he asked the Academia Mexicana to sponsor an International Congress on Traditional and Folk Medicine. This congress has been a great success, with annual meetings that attract over a thousand participants and observers, all of whom share an interest in the subject of traditional medicine. Much of the identification, chemical analysis, and research into the uses of medicinal herbs in Mexico and Latin America is done by the participants in this international congress. Presenters come from thirty different countries and represent a variety of disciplines, including anthropology, ethnology, ecology, and a broad variety of health-care specializations, including curanderismo. This interdisciplinary approach to the study of traditional medicine is unique in its breadth and helps foster a much better understanding of what the various disciplines can bring to the study of traditional approaches to health care. The congress has hosted eleven international and five national gatherings.

Although Mexico has the largest population of curanderos of any country in Latin America, Dr. Hutterer realized that countries such as Peru, Bolivia, India, and China were more advanced in traditional medicine than Mexico was. Also, the curanderos in Mexico had no recognized voice or meeting place. Thanks to the Academia Mexicana, Dr. Hutterer has united many folk healers in his country as well as many healers from all over the world. "We have to learn to respect the curandero and to recognize him as a colleague. We need to learn from him. Medical doctors are very ignorant of popular medicine and folk medicine, and I learned that my education was not focused on the people I serve. Western doctors are in error when all they focus on is 'advancement' and ignore the ancestors. I learned that modern medicine is a system based on a technological market that favors a few. They treat the rich. The poor cannot afford this system."

When I asked Dr. Hutterer why he did not become a curandero, he said, "I *am* a curandero. A curandero is a healer who has the vocation and the *don*." When I asked him what he thought of as the future of curanderismo, his response was encouraging and inspiring: "My vision is that all medicines become one, and that many curative methods will exist as complementary medicines. My future as a doctor should be to solve my pueblo's illness with a curandero next to me. We are complementary. I want to work hand in hand with technicians, traditional practitioners, and scientists."

In recent years, Dr. Hutterer has initiated an international award for practitioners, researchers, and others who have contributed to the advancement of traditional and folk medicine. Since 1991, the Martin de la Cruz Medal has been awarded to forty people worldwide. Martin de la Cruz was an Aztec physician who wrote the first book on the Aztec's use of medicinal herbs and translated it into Castillian Spanish. Dr. Eliseo Torres, Ehekateotl, Andres Segura, and I have all received this prestigious award.

Tieraona Low Dog: M.D. and Herbalist

While Dr. Tieraona Low Dog is not a curandera, she is another of the new breed of health-care professionals who have earned medical degrees at universities yet have not abandoned the folk medicine of their roots. While growing up at the Standing Rock Reservation in South Dakota, Dr. Low Dog always assumed that everyone used herbs in treating illness. By watching the medicine people work, she learned early on that many sicknesses result from sadness and pain in the soul, which her Lakota tribe calls "ghost sickness," and that a healthy body results from a well-balanced soul and spirit. Dr. Low Dog says, "We try to heal the body. We don't pay a lot of attention to the soul, which is sad, because Western medicine's roots were very much in the religious."

Even though she is now a practicing M.D., Dr. Low Dog has not abandoned the use of herbs. Long before she decided to go to medical school, she gathered, grew, and prescribed herbs to people in her community at Standing Rock. The first time she wrote out a prescription for antibiotics as a physician, she was struck by the disturbing fact that she didn't know anything about the drug she was prescribing. She realized that she'd never taken it, didn't know where it came from or under what kind of conditions it had been grown or produced, whether it had been tested on animals, or how carefully it had been prepared. She also realized that a good many of the low-income families that she sees at the University of New Mexico Family Practice Clinic where she works have difficulty affording the drugs that most doctors prescribe. For this reason, she educates them on the uses of a few basic herbs, and tells them how to prepare tinctures so that they can avoid the expense of buying them in a health-food store.

Especially during cold and flu season, she encourages parents to give their families a tincture of echinacea, which has been clinically proven to strengthen the immune system. This herb is safe for practically everyone, including children, because it has no toxicity, no lethal dose, and no side-effects. It can even be taken during pregnancy and lactation. She also suggests that some patients suffering from depression try St. John's wort, which is a natural antidepressant. This herb takes effect in three to four weeks, has no effect on cardiac conductivity, and no side-effects such as sexual dysfunction. Both echinacea and St. John's wort are herbs that have been clinically well tested, and are routinely prescribed by French and German doctors.

Aside from herbs, Dr. Low Dog uses a variety of tools to heal her patients, such as meditation, and wellness visits for the terminally ill during which they are forbidden to mention their illness. "If the only way you can go to a doctor is if you're sick, then, strange as it may seem, there's a motivation to always remain ill." She looks at every encounter with patients as an opportunity to explore their feelings as well as their physical symptoms. While she feels that Western doctors have diagnoses down pat, she feels they have a long way to go when it really comes to knowing how to treat people, body and soul. Her dream is to staff hospital waiting rooms and emergency rooms with grandmothers who can sit with those who are waiting to see doctors, because these elders know how to ask people the right questions, reassure parents who are concerned and upset, and comfort children who are ill.

One of the things she finds so fascinating about her patients is the language that they use to describe their ailments—and the kind of language she must learn to be able to communicate with them medically. For example, she has found that if you ask many Hispanic people if they are depressed, they will answer "No." This is especially true of older Hispanic men, who consider depression a character failing. However, if you ask these same individuals if they are having problems sleeping, if their appetite is poor, or if they are feeling sad, many of them will say "Yes." She also discovered that people who would not take an antidepressant if she offered it to them would respond if she said, "Here is an herb that just might lift your spirits."

Her patients seek her out, she believes, because she has a foot in both doors, in modern medicine and in folk medicine. She recalls one instance when she helped a family through the difficult act of taking their father, Nestor, off his life-support equipment. When it became clear that Nestor was not going to make it, she asked his two sons when they wanted to disconnect him from the equipment. When they told her they wanted to do so the next morning, the other doctors at the hospital complained. "This machine costs eight thousand dollars a day," they said. Dr. Low Dog insisted that the hospital wait because she felt that the matter concerned people's hearts, not cold dollars and cents.

She asked the sons to bring in pictures of their father and his favorite music, which she put in a tape player. She then drew the curtains around the intensive care unit, and asked the sons if they wanted to talk about their father. They told her how well liked he was in his little town. When they were finally ready, she asked the nurses to turn off all the bells and buzzers, then she disconnected the machine and gently let Nestor go. "Would you like us to pray together, or would you like to be left alone to cry?" she asked the sons. They asked her to pray with them, and the three of them joined hands next to the father's bed. Everyone in the ward said that a beautiful spirit of peace remained in that intensive care unit for the rest of the day. "Even though I was not a member of the sons' culture," said Low Dog, "we were able to share the sacredness of this together, because we are all just people."

Back when I was working as a nurse, there were so many times when I wanted to bring curanderismo and spirituality into the hospital setting, but I wasn't allowed. As a nurse, I had even less power than a doctor. For me, I had to leave the institution, but I am very happy that today people like Dr. Low Dog are able to fight to keep the medicine of the people in modern hospitals. Dr. Low Dog gives me hope when she reports that, even though her medical training was brutal, and that many well-intentioned men and women do not make it through medical school with their souls intact, she is thankful that she was somehow able to remain faithful to her ideal. When I speak to doctors such as her, I realize freshly that many complex, highly effective, heart-centered medical systems existed long before there were medical schools.

Integrated Medicine for the "World Family"

Over the last ten years, as I have begun to participate more and more in conferences that focus on gathering together folk practitioners from around the world, I have come in contact with some extraordinary organizations dedicated to exploring and bringing together traditional healers from many cultures. One of the groups from which I have learned a great deal is the Center for Natural and Traditional Medicines, located in Washington, D.C. CNTM was cofounded by Kaiya Montaocean, John Rutayuga, and Vera Pratt. Montaocean is a woman of mixed Irish and Apache descent raised on an Indian reservation in Oklahoma; John Rutayuga is an advocate for integrated global health care whose mother had been a traditional healer; and Vera Pratt has a background in environmental studies and community activism. CNTM is dedicated to the preservation and promotion of indigenous traditional medical knowledge, so that these practices can be used as the basis of an integrated and sustainable global health-care program.

Over the years I have become very close with Kaiya Montaocean. I first met her in 1988 when she invited me to participate in the first national conference on alternative and complementary therapies. At the time, there was no existing network of folk practitioners and researchers, so she found me through word of mouth. People told her that there was a woman somewhere in the Southwest who was advocating that curanderismo provided a great foundation for community-based care. When Kaiya first approached the conference's organizing committee, which was heavily composed of modern medical doctors and academics, about incorporating people like me into the conference, they were skeptical. Alternative medicine was okay, but folk medicine—well, that was iffy. They said, "Maybe we can have one or two people like her at the conference, but we have no scientific evidence supporting the failure or success of folk practitioners."

Kaiya, however, was determined to involve health-care

practitioners from every segment of the society. On her own, she raised funds to include not only me but African American, African Caribbean, Native American, East Indian, Asian, and African folk practitioners. The conference, which was held at Walter Reed Hospital in Washington, D.C., was a great success, and the folk practitioners really opened the eyes of the other participants, who, in 1988, were deeply involved in developing the fields of alternative medicine. What was so exciting for the alternative practitioners was that, for the first time, many of them were able to connect directly with the roots of their practices. This was a beautiful and necessary reunion.

The center's growing support for regional conferences and discussions led to its involvement in working with a variety of organizations around the world, including the African Holistic Health Association, the Indian Health Services, the Chinese Healing Arts Institute, and the Academia Mexicana de Medicina Tradicional, in their forums and symposiums. Today CNTM has created an organization called the Healing Roots Network, which promotes communication among a consortium of individuals and nongovernmental organizations (NGOs) that work on how to integrate natural and traditional medicines along with appropriate technology throughout the world. Kaiya reports: "As of this date, we are actively supporting the establishment and implementation of grassroots Traditional Medicine and Environment Centers in South Africa, Senegal, Nigeria, Ghana, Thailand, Mongolia, India, Peru, Ecuador, Brazil, Chile, El Salvador, Guatemala, Belize, Jamaica, Surinam, and among the sovereign native nations in North America including the Seminole, Apache, Kiowa, Comanche, Cherokee, Diné (Navaho), and Hopi.

"The goal of the Healing Roots Network is to reawaken the people's consciousness to the reality that our ancestral medicines and the knowledge that they left us is not dead or extinct but alive and thriving in most of the communities around our Mother Earth. It is up to us to cherish it and re-organize it into an accessible knowledge base and network so that it can be connected beyond the artificial border of nation states. The healing arts are a global phenomenon and every group, every culture, has a color, an image, a brushstroke to add to the ever-growing mural of therapies and cures."

One of the points that Kaiya stresses is that, while modern medical doctors look down on alternative medicine, an astonishing 80 percent of the world's people use some form of folk or alternative treatment, even though ethnic groups in the U.S. have much fear and shame about openly discussing their use of traditional medicines. The irony is that while this denial and criticism of folk and alternative medicines is going on, the mainstream health-care system in the United States is literally falling apart. But Kaiya believes that this disintegration of the status quo offers us hope. "When things fall apart we are really able to look inside and make the necessary changes."

Kaiya's vision of the future of curanderismo and traditional medicines is very similar to my own. "Because these are medicines of the heart, they are leading us into the center to re-envision and re-create a health system that is a circle where all people can belong. It is a circle that will not minimize the importance of plentiful organic food, medicinal plants, clean water, clean air, and affordable and appropriate technology."

New Plants Out of Old Roots

During my parents' generation, the fires of racism burned over the ground of our culture, creating shame, denial of our heritage and customs, and the pressure to assimilate. But now, out of this scorched earth, new plants are growing from the roots of those that had been burned. Like precious seeds that went into hiding, curanderismo is being reborn within me and within a new generation of young women to whom I am now teaching this medicine.

One of the most wonderful things about curanderismo is that it is a direct expression of the personality of the practitioner. Although I am a very traditional curandera who uses the *plática*, performs *limpias* using the egg, and does soul retrievals, yet my dramatic, passionate nature is very much in evidence in my work. As my students have begun to utilize curanderismo in their own work, I have seen how much each woman has drawn on and expressed the essence of who she truly is. While most of them cannot bring this medicine into their jobs in its pure form, I am constantly impressed and touched by how creative they are in utilizing curanderismo's spirit in their interactions with their patients and clients. To me, this kind of weaving, this kind of mindfulness, represents the future of curanderismo, which expresses itself in their work as loving concern, compassion, patience, creativity, soul awareness, and self-awareness. Here are a few of their stories showing how they have taken this medicine and made it their own.

Irene, whose Nahuatl name is Coatl, works at the middle management level for a large state agency in Santa Fe. Because of her agency's closeness to the seat of state government, she finds that the conservative political currents in the capital tend to stifle any framework of thought that differs from the mainstream. In addition, unlike many of my apprentices, who are either nurses or body workers of some kind, Irene does not work with individual patients but with clinical directors and their staffs at nonprofit agencies contracted to provide services to children and their families. As a result, she has to be very creative in utilizing the principles of curanderismo in her workplace. Nevertheless she has found a number of interesting ways to apply the spiritual, philosophical, and cultural lessons that she has learned.

On the personal level, she takes the time to "listen from the heart to colleagues in need of a 'mini-*plática*.' I also open the meetings that I facilitate with an invocation to the Creator. I have asked people from various traditions to perform a ritual from their culture at the beginning of these meetings. When this happens, I notice that the participants are calmer, listen better, and are more open to one another. They seem to speak in a more heartfelt way, and everyone has expressed the desire to continue to open the meetings with a sacred moment."

Irene also uses curanderismo to help her to cope with the day-to-day stresses of the work environment. "When I personally sustain a work-related *susto*, I have learned to achieve a renewed sense of balance and peace by smudging myself with copal smoke after work."

Curanderismo has helped Irene to create a greater outreach into the communities that she works with. She has asked healers from the Native American programs that she comes in contact with through her work if they would be interested in participating in the upcoming Congress of Tradi-

tional Medicine, which will be held in Albuquerque in 1998.
So far, all have said yes. Irene's future work with curanderismo will include ways to utilize its principles into work
with youth at risk. "I hope to integrate a series of *pláticas* by
Ehekateotl into a program serving youth who have been sus-
pended from school. Ehe's message of knowing your place in
the universe, your connection to your ancestors and to history, and acting in accord with the universal principles of
equilibrium will be empowering and healing for these youth."

Valerie (Cuetzpalin) has been a Rolfer for ten years, and
works with her clients' muscular and emotional holding patterns. Although she doesn't use curanderismo in her work directly unless the client asks for it, she is fascinated with the
parallels she sees between the two treatment modalities.
"When one reads the writings of Ida Rolf, many of her ideas
reflect concepts of curanderismo. Both Rolfers and curanderos are taught how to really listen in a *plática* for a person's
needs beyond what they are even saying." When Valerie
works with a client she watches him "using my vision and intuition to see various mannerisms, habits, and fixations in the
bodily expression. In curanderismo, one is doing this and
more. We really enter into the history and reality of the person in both areas. When someone finally comes to be Rolfed,
he is here for a change in some way, whether he is suffering
from physical pain, emotional trauma, abuse, or the simple
desire for more mobility or wanting to be more present in his
body. The added richness of curanderismo validates what I
have already felt and intuited in my work, and adds even
more dimensions to what affects a person's health.

"One client named Sara was about to be married for the

third time. Her last marriage had been abusive and she expressed a deep need to move on, leaving those abusive patterns behind. She could feel them in the ways that the energy in her body was contracted in various places, tightening her voice, her guts, her chest, and her breathing. Sara spoke a lot about spirit and the need for ceremony and ritual, so I offered her a prewedding *limpia*. She came with all kinds of pictures and objects related to her past marriages, and many objects associated with her mother, who she felt was holding on to her in a negative and dependent way. During the ceremony, Sara did a lot of letting go, finally admitting her part in creating all of these life events. By the time we came to the *limpia*, she was able to clearly express her need to separate from her mother in order to have a healthy marriage. During the *limpia*, I was able to add in the Rolfing, helping her to let go physically. The physical, emotional, mental, and spiritual aspects of her health were all being addressed."

Pat (Xochitl) is a registered nurse who is currently managing a sixty-six unit apartment complex in Paradise Hills, New Mexico. A lot of spousal abuse and violence goes on in some of these units, and when a family moves out, Pat does a house blessing and cleansing before the new tenant moves in. She waits until the place is completely cleaned, painted, and recarpeted, then takes her copal and candles, purifies each room of all negative energies, and then blesses the house to make it ready for the next tenant. "I take this work very seriously because I want to provide people with a peaceful place to live." She is even keeping records to see if the apartments that have been cleansed and blessed have a lower turnover rate than the other units. Most important, she is taking to heart curanderismo's belief that a sense of community is one of the foundations of health. She puts a tremendous amount of energy into planting special trees, providing her tenants with outdoor places to relax, and offering recreational outlets such as basketball hoops for the kids. Since she has begun this work, she has seen a marked improvement in the energy of the apartment complex and in the renters themselves.

Soledad (Ehecatl) is a professional art photographer who exhibits in galleries and museums. For years she has been taking self-portraits, creating the setting, stepping in front of the camera, and intuitively taking the picture. "For years, I didn't know why I was so driven to photograph myself and why it was so easy for me to do it. That has become clear to me since studying with Elena. I didn't realize that I was allowing bits of my soul to be seen and heard through these images. The moment I step from behind the camera into the small world I've created in front of the camera, I let intuition take over completely. I listen to my soul and trust that magic will happen. It usually does. As I have learned through Elena and Ehekateotl, one must always confront the smoky gray mirror. I had been doing that for years through my work. Now I have an opportunity to practice doing it in all aspects of my life."

Recently Soledad has come up with the idea of using her photography skills as a kind of visual curanderismo to help people catch glimpses of their own souls. "For years, people have asked me to photograph them as I do myself. In the past I had been reluctant. I wasn't sure that I could get people to open up enough to create an image that revealed more than just the surface. Studying with Elena has given me the confidence and the desire to [do so]. I am presently taking such images of other people. In the future I would like to take them a step further by offering . . . a *plática*, perhaps a soul retrieval, and then an image. [These tools] are a way to open up and prepare the person to be photographed, to be vulnerable enough to let their intuitive nature take over. This kind of image becomes an X-ray of the soul. . . . I have always accepted the notion that it was possible to absorb [information] without cognitive questioning, believing that understanding was a process that would form itself. This is at the root of curanderismo."

Elise (Atl), a nurse and street outreach worker, cautions that although some people desperately need what curanderismo has to offer, it is important to be sensitive to their receptivity to treatment. This is a challenging task for the healer, whose perceptions and insights often awaken her compassion and her desire to be of service. "I had the chance to give a *limpia* to a patient with AIDS. In addition to having some brain damage from huffing (sniffing paint and other volatile substances), this fellow was also a chronic inventor of stories. Lying seems to be a huge symptom of addiction. He probably has some AIDS-related dementia too. Anyhow, this fellow was rarely taken seriously by most of his caregivers, and thus his emotional needs surrounding his AIDS diagnosis were rarely, if ever, met. There is a pretty thick, tough-guy patina on this fellow. I had known him for years and asked him one day if he would like a *limpia*. He declined, despite my effort to explain the benefits. I really wanted to do this for him, an alternative healing approach that I knew in my heart would help. Yet, as someone who has been a caregiver for over two decades, I feel that I probably pushed too hard. You can't help someone who isn't ready to be helped."

Alice (Ozomatl) worked as a child-development specialist for eighteen years and has been a professional massage therapist for three years. Curanderismo taught her "the sense of community, of caring for and helping each other." Recently she had an opportunity to help her father, who has been struggling with cancer. Her father is a man who grew up with folk medicine, rejected it in favor of modern medicine, but is starting once again to accept help from the old ways. Recently when Alice visited him in the hospital, he allowed her to do ceremony with him. Afterward he told her that "his spirit lifted after the ceremony, a heavy darkness lifted up." This experience reminded Alice of her grandmother, Nene, a skilled curandera whom people referred to as La Señora, the Queen of the Mountain. People always called for her grandmother when they were sick in the hospital, and Nene's healing presence always brought peace. It took courage for Alice to offer the gifts of curanderismo to her father, but she intuitively knew it was the right thing to do. Both she and her father received a great sense of peace from the experience.

Lorraine (Ocelotl) is a nurse practitioner who works for an HMO. She finds this environment frustrating because patients are seen as "customers" and only allowed fifteen minutes of her time or the doctor's time. "Presently a big percentage of the people I see on a daily basis have many physical complaints. I believe many of these people are in physical pain with an underlying depression, which I believe comes from many years of mental anguish, in other words, soul loss." Some of her patients who know that she is studying curanderismo have asked her to give them *limpias*, but she has referred them to her comadres. In her present situation at the HMO, she feels that inviting these patients to her home for treatment would be considered a conflict of interest. "Of course, I will lay my hands on those patients whom I have a good rapport with and give them a short massage, especially those who break down crying because of home situations — marital conflict, and physical, emotional, and sexual abuse. We will exchange conversation focusing on depression, self-care, feelings of loss, and the possibility of soul loss. I share some of my own experiences with them, which always seems to give them courage to open up even more about themselves. This is considered *unprofessional* in our present-day system. These patients are usually Hispanic, Mexican, or Anglo women who have had some exposure to similar types of treatment. Of course, the society we live in, which allows the clock to run our lives, does not help matters any. The push to see patients in a very short time does not allow for further treatment. I end up having to refer them to a therapist."

Lorraine's dream is eventually to have a health clinic where she and her comadres can pool their various skills and talents and put them to use serving the people. In the future she would like to be able to see patients in one- or two-hour sessions, enabling her to do thorough *pláticas*, *limpias*, and soul retrievals. She also plans on becoming certified in phytotherapy (the uses of herbs) and massage therapy.

Jeri (Cozcacuáuhtli) is a psychiatric nurse who works with teenaged boys from troubled family backgrounds. These young kids have developed thick skins and ways to hide their feelings as a means of survival. To Jeri the wilderness is the place to heal, and she often takes groups of young boys out into the woods for overnight trips. To her the wilderness is the place of "deep peace, the place where healing occurs. In the wild all parts of each of us are exposed, illuminated, and honored." One of the tools of curanderismo that she uses is the talking circle. "We use this circle as a way of relating, sorting, integrating, and staying connected. Each person's voice strengthens the power of the community as the teacher becomes the student and the student becomes the teacher. . . . Sharing our own stories and listening really creates a sacred space. So much work is done in these *pláticas*. Working with the energy as it emerges it like opening blinded eyes to the beauty that is our legacy, and a part of the healing medicine.

"One night in early fall on an expedition far up into Beaver Creek, we had completed our talking circle later than usual and had settled under our tarps as ice was already forming in our water bottles. Suddenly a young boy's cries, shrill and piercing, exploded from the next tarp. 'Get up, get up right now and get out here. Hurry.' I was out of my bag in one barefooted leap, expecting an emergency, only to find him standing in the field, arms outstretched, head back. 'Look at the stars, just look at the stars,' he said. Although I've stopped predicting when healing will begin, I do recognize the moment. This boy's face was a reflection of that energy."

An Ancient Medicine Lives On

For me it is so gratifying to hear the stories of my students, to see the seeds of curanderismo sprout and make such beautiful flowers and strong plants. This medicine is growing and changing, reaching out and forming new pathways for its expression. The roots are strong, and the new growth is getting stronger. When I was told by my teacher Ehekateotl that I would be accountable for these women for the rest of my life, it seemed like a big responsibility, but I also know that it's one that I have always wanted. I've always wanted other people to see the beauty of curanderismo. These students are the reflection of what I've taught them. Not only are they using curanderismo to be of service to others within their communities and their workplaces but they are also giving their families the benefits. When Soledad's son lost his half brother, she led him through a ceremony to help him grieve. Alice's father requests *limpias* from his daughter to deal with his cancer. Valerie climbs into bed with her dying mother and holds her all night. One day my apprentices will also be teachers who will pass the medicine on to their children and their students.

I'm happy to be able to stand in the direction of the north and tell my ancestors that I did not let this medicine die. To me, curanderismo is the art of creating beauty, culture, and medicine with all the power and imagination of the curandera's spirit and soul. Perhaps my destiny was unfolding even as a child when I stole the flowers that I needed for my ceremonies. To the ancient Aztecs, "flower and song" meant poetry—seeking the truth through the pursuit of art and beauty. The healing art of curanderismo possesses a variety of flowers, fragrant plants to feed the spirit and body, hundreds of *yerbas buenas*—good herbs, candles flickering with the prayers and wishes that light our path, the sounds of the eagle feather sweeping away despair and *mal aire*, delivering these sorrows to Iztacmixcoatl, the Serpent of White Clouds. Curanderismo embraces the sounds of music, songs, drumming, and chants that release the blocked places, the *empacho* in our hearts and bodies. It is the medicine of loving hands that untwist the knots within envious hearts, and loving voices filled with laughter that unstop the backflow of our *bilis,* our rage. When the curandera calls out the name of your soul, she helps you to return to your true nature, which the Aztecs called "face and heart." As she sweeps something as simple as an egg made sacred by pure intent over your body, she helps free you from troubling, tormenting thoughts and from the energy that does not belong to you.

I do not want to hoard the life-giving medicine of curanderismo but to share it freely with all who are willing to listen. Rediscovering these sacred roots of my culture was a long and arduous journey. To find the buried seeds and nuggets of curanderismo—that name that includes ideas of priest, curing, and caring, all in one word—I personally had to unearth the metaphorical remains of my grandparents. I fear that my soul would still be wandering lost and neglected if I had not reclaimed and reunited with the curandera within me. I now spread the seeds to my global family, the animated spirit of the many serpent heads of all the world's continents, the rainbow serpents that glow in the dark.

My prayers to Coyolxauhqui, the Cosmic Mother, have been answered as I release this book to my cosmic family. Because I have lived long enough to see my future generations, I have truly lived enough to die. It is my hope that the luminous science of curanderismo will live as long as the earth lives, and will continue to grind our pain into seeds that sleep through the winter of our sorrow while we wait patiently for new seedlings to appear—tender shoots, tiny-fisted leaves, so green with youth, so old with love.

Index

About the Authors

A registered nurse with a master's degree in psychiatric nursing, for twenty-five years **Elena Avila** has been a professional curandera practicing traditional Mexican/Chicano folk medicine. An international speaker and workshop presenter on curanderismo, Avila lives in New Mexico.

Joy Parker is an ethnographic writer who has taught at Columbia University and New York University. She is the coauthor of *A Forest of Kings: The Untold Story of the Ancient Maya* and *Maya Cosmos*.